Cardiology Simplified

Understanding Heart Health
and Advanced Cardiac
Treatments

Sydney Dean

loss due to the information herein, either directly or indirectly. Respective authors own all copyrights not held by the publisher. The information herein is offered for informational purposes solely, and is universal as so. The presentation of the information is without contract or any type of guarantee assurance. The trademarks that are used are without any consent, and the publication of the trademark is without permission or backing by the trademark owner. All trademarks and brands within this book are for clarifying purposes only and are the owned by the owners themselves, not affiliated with this document.

Table of Contents

Chapter 1

Introduction to Cardiology

What is Cardiology?

Cardiology is the branch of medicine that deals with the diagnosis, treatment, and prevention of diseases and disorders of the heart and blood vessels. As a specialized field, it encompasses a wide range of conditions, procedures, and technologies aimed at maintaining and restoring the health of one of the body's most vital organs. Understanding cardiology is crucial for anyone interested in heart health, whether they are medical professionals, patients, or simply individuals looking to take proactive steps towards a healthier lifestyle.

Cardiology has a rich history that stretches back centuries, with roots in ancient civilizations such as Egypt and Greece. Early physicians like Hippocrates and Galen made significant contributions to understanding the heart, even if their theories were rudimentary by today's standards. The true evolution of cardiac care began in the Renaissance period when anatomists like Andreas Vesalius started to systematically study human anatomy. However, it wasn't until the 20th century that cardiology emerged as a distinct medical specialty, driven by technological advancements and groundbreaking research.

The heart, a powerful muscular organ roughly the size of a fist, is responsible for pumping blood throughout the body, supplying oxygen and nutrients to tissues, and removing carbon dioxide and other wastes. It functions tirelessly, beating approximately 100,000 times a day and moving about 5 liters of blood per minute. This relentless activity underscores the importance of heart health, as even minor disruptions can have significant ramifications for overall well-being.

Heart health is crucial for maintaining the body's homeostasis. The heart's ability to efficiently pump blood ensures that all bodily systems receive the oxygen and nutrients they need to function optimally. When the heart is compromised, it can lead to a cascade of health issues, affecting everything from energy levels and cognitive function to immune response and longevity. Thus, cardiology plays a vital role in identifying, treating, and preventing conditions that can impair heart function.

Common heart conditions include coronary artery disease (CAD), heart failure, arrhythmias, and valvular heart diseases. Each of these conditions presents unique challenges and requires specific diagnostic and therapeutic approaches. For instance, CAD, the most common type of heart disease, is characterized by the buildup of plaque in the coronary arteries, which can lead to heart attacks if left untreated. Heart failure, on the other hand, occurs when the heart is unable to pump blood effectively, leading to symptoms like shortness of breath, fatigue, and fluid retention.

Arrhythmias, or irregular heartbeats, can range from benign to life-threatening. They occur when the electrical impulses that coordinate heartbeats are disrupted, causing the heart to beat too fast, too slow, or erratically. Valvular heart diseases involve damage or defects in one or more of the heart's valves, which can affect blood flow and lead to complications like heart failure or stroke. Understanding these conditions is fundamental for both preventing and managing heart disease.

Cardiac treatments have advanced significantly over the years, offering patients a variety of options to manage and overcome heart conditions. These treatments can be broadly categorized into lifestyle modifications, medications, and surgical interventions. Lifestyle modifications, such as adopting a heart-healthy diet, engaging in regular physical activity, and avoiding smoking, are foundational strategies for maintaining heart health and preventing disease progression. These changes can significantly reduce the risk of heart disease and improve outcomes for those already diagnosed with heart conditions.

Medications play a crucial role in managing heart disease. For instance, statins are commonly prescribed to lower cholesterol levels, reducing the risk of plaque buildup in the arteries. Beta-blockers and ACE inhibitors are used to manage blood pressure and heart failure, while anticoagulants and antiplatelet drugs help prevent blood clots that can lead to heart attacks or strokes. Advances in pharmacology have led to the development of newer drugs that offer more effective management of heart conditions with fewer side effects.

Surgical interventions are often necessary when lifestyle changes and medications are insufficient. Procedures like angioplasty and stent placement can open blocked arteries, restoring blood flow to the heart. Coronary artery bypass grafting (CABG) is another common procedure that involves creating a bypass around blocked arteries using vessels from other parts of the body. For patients with severe heart valve disease, valve repair or replacement surgery may be required. In cases of advanced heart failure, heart transplantation or the use of mechanical assist devices might be considered.

Preventive cardiology focuses on identifying and mitigating risk factors for heart disease before they lead to serious health issues. This proactive approach involves regular screenings and assessments to detect early signs of heart disease, allowing for timely intervention. Preventive strategies also emphasize the importance of managing chronic conditions like hypertension, diabetes, and high cholesterol, which are significant risk factors for heart disease.

Education and awareness are integral components of cardiology. By understanding the risk factors and early warning signs of heart disease, individuals can take steps to protect their heart health. Regular check-ups with healthcare providers, adherence to prescribed treatments, and lifestyle modifications are key elements of a heart-healthy regimen. Public health initiatives and educational campaigns aim to raise awareness about heart disease and promote behaviors that support cardiovascular health.

The future of cardiology looks promising, with ongoing research and technological advancements paving the way for new treatments and improved patient outcomes. Innovations such as personalized medicine, which tailors treatments to an individual's genetic makeup, and regenerative therapies, which aim to repair damaged heart tissue, hold great potential. Additionally, advancements in imaging and diagnostic tools are enhancing our ability to detect and treat heart disease at earlier stages.

Historical Evolution of Cardiac Care

Cardiac care has undergone a remarkable transformation over the centuries, evolving from rudimentary understandings and treatments to highly sophisticated and specialized medical practices. The journey of this evolution is marked by significant milestones, breakthroughs, and the relentless pursuit of knowledge, driven by the desire to understand and combat heart disease.

In ancient civilizations, the heart was often considered the seat of emotion and life force. Early Egyptian and Greek physicians made some of the first documented attempts to understand cardiac function. The Ebers Papyrus, an ancient Egyptian medical text dating back to around 1550 BCE, contains references to heart diseases and treatments, albeit limited in scope and scientific accuracy. Similarly, Greek physician Hippocrates, often regarded as the father of medicine, made observations about the heart's role in the circulatory system, though his theories were largely speculative.

Galen, a prominent Greek physician of the Roman era, made significant strides in the anatomical understanding of the heart. His work in the second century AD, based on animal dissections, offered insights into the heart's structure and function.

However, many of his theories, such as the belief that blood was produced in the liver and consumed by the body, were later proven incorrect. Despite these inaccuracies, Galen's influence persisted for centuries, shaping early medical thought.

The Renaissance period marked a pivotal shift in the understanding of cardiac anatomy and physiology. Andreas Vesalius, a Flemish anatomist, challenged Galenic doctrine through meticulous human dissections. His seminal work, "De humani corporis fabrica" (On the Fabric of the Human Body), published in 1543, provided detailed and accurate depictions of the heart and its vessels. This work laid the foundation for modern anatomy and inspired further exploration into the cardiovascular system.

William Harvey, an English physician, made one of the most groundbreaking discoveries in the history of cardiac care. In 1628, he published "De Motu Cordis" (On the Motion of the Heart and Blood), where he described the systemic circulation of blood and the heart's role as a pump. Harvey's meticulous experiments and observations demonstrated that blood circulates continuously through the body in a closed system of vessels, revolutionizing medical understanding and debunking centuries-old misconceptions.

The 19th century witnessed rapid advancements in medical science, significantly influencing cardiac

care. The invention of the stethoscope by René
Laennec in 1816 allowed physicians to auscultate
heart sounds, providing a non-invasive method to
diagnose heart conditions. This period also saw the
development of the sphygmomanometer by Samuel
Siegfried Karl Ritter von Basch in 1881, enabling
accurate measurement of blood pressure—a critical
factor in assessing cardiovascular health.

The advent of the 20th century heralded an era of
unprecedented progress in cardiology. Technological
innovations, coupled with a deeper understanding of
cardiac physiology and pathology, led to the
development of new diagnostic and therapeutic
techniques. Willem Einthoven's invention of the
electrocardiogram (ECG) in 1903 revolutionized
cardiac diagnostics by allowing the electrical activity
of the heart to be recorded and analyzed. This
breakthrough enabled the identification of various
cardiac abnormalities, such as arrhythmias and
myocardial infarctions, with greater precision.

The mid-20th century saw the emergence of cardiac
catheterization, pioneered by German physician
Werner Forssmann in 1929. By threading a catheter
into his own heart, Forssmann demonstrated a
technique that would become fundamental in
diagnosing and treating heart conditions. Cardiac
catheterization allowed for direct measurement of
intracardiac pressures and visualization of the

coronary arteries, paving the way for interventional cardiology.

The development of open-heart surgery marked another monumental leap in cardiac care. In 1953, John Gibbon successfully performed the first open-heart surgery using a heart-lung machine, which maintained circulation and oxygenation during the procedure. This innovation made it possible to correct congenital and acquired heart defects that were previously considered inoperable. Subsequent advancements in surgical techniques, such as coronary artery bypass grafting (CABG) and heart valve replacement, further expanded the therapeutic arsenal available to cardiac surgeons.

Pharmacological advancements have also played a crucial role in the evolution of cardiac care. The discovery and development of drugs to manage heart disease have significantly improved patient outcomes. For example, the introduction of beta-blockers in the 1960s provided a powerful tool to manage hypertension and arrhythmias. Similarly, the development of statins in the 1980s revolutionized the treatment of hyperlipidemia, reducing the risk of coronary artery disease.

The late 20th and early 21st centuries have seen the advent of minimally invasive procedures, offering patients safer and less traumatic alternatives to traditional surgery. Percutaneous coronary intervention (PCI), commonly known as angioplasty, allows for the dilation of narrowed coronary arteries using a balloon catheter. The subsequent placement of stents helps maintain vessel patency, reducing the need for more invasive surgical interventions. Similarly, transcatheter aortic valve replacement (TAVR) provides a less invasive option for patients with severe aortic stenosis who are at high risk for open-heart surgery.

Advances in imaging technology have further enhanced our ability to diagnose and treat heart disease. Techniques such as echocardiography, cardiac magnetic resonance imaging (MRI), and computed tomography (CT) angiography provide detailed images of the heart's structure and function. These non-invasive imaging modalities allow for early detection of cardiac abnormalities, guiding treatment decisions and improving patient outcomes.

The field of electrophysiology has also seen significant advancements, particularly in the management of arrhythmias. The development of implantable devices such as pacemakers and defibrillators has revolutionized the treatment of life-threatening heart rhythm disorders. Catheter ablation, a procedure that destroys or isolates areas of the heart responsible for abnormal electrical signals, offers a curative option for many patients with arrhythmias.

In recent years, the integration of digital technology and data analytics has opened new frontiers in cardiac care. Wearable devices and remote monitoring systems enable continuous tracking of heart health, providing real-time data that can inform personalized treatment plans. Artificial intelligence and machine learning algorithms are being developed to analyze vast amounts of data, potentially identifying patterns and predicting cardiac events before they occur.

Importance of Heart Health

The heart, a remarkable organ roughly the size of a fist, is the engine that drives the human body. It pumps oxygenated blood to vital organs and tissues, sustaining life and facilitating the myriad functions that keep us alive and thriving. Understanding the importance of heart health is crucial not only for medical professionals but for everyone, as the well-being of our heart directly impacts our overall health and longevity.

Heart disease is one of the leading causes of death globally, claiming millions of lives each year. This stark reality underscores the critical need to prioritize heart health. Heart disease encompasses a range of conditions, including coronary artery disease, heart failure, arrhythmias, and valvular heart diseases. Each of these conditions can significantly impair quality of life and, if left untreated, can be fatal. Therefore, maintaining heart health is not just about living longer but also about living better.

One of the foundational aspects of heart health is understanding and managing risk factors. Some risk factors, such as age, sex, and family history, are beyond our control. However, many others are modifiable through lifestyle changes and medical interventions. High blood pressure, high cholesterol, smoking, obesity, physical inactivity, and diabetes are among the most significant modifiable risk factors. By addressing these, individuals can substantially reduce their risk of developing heart disease.

High blood pressure, or hypertension, is often called the "silent killer" because it typically has no symptoms until significant damage has occurred. It puts extra strain on the heart and blood vessels, increasing the risk of heart attacks, strokes, and heart failure. Regular monitoring and management of blood pressure through lifestyle changes, such as reducing salt intake, maintaining a healthy weight, and exercising regularly, are vital. In some cases, medication may be necessary to keep blood pressure within a healthy range.

Cholesterol, a fatty substance found in the blood, is essential for building healthy cells. However, high levels of low-density lipoprotein (LDL) cholesterol can lead to the buildup of plaques in the arteries, a condition known as atherosclerosis. This can restrict blood flow and lead to heart attacks and strokes. Lifestyle changes, such as eating a heart-healthy diet low in saturated and trans fats, exercising regularly, and quitting smoking, can help manage cholesterol levels. For some individuals, medications such as statins may be required to reduce cholesterol effectively.

Smoking is one of the most significant risk factors for heart disease. The chemicals in tobacco smoke damage the heart and blood vessels, leading to the narrowing of arteries (atherosclerosis), increased blood pressure, and reduced oxygen in the blood. Quitting smoking is one of the best things individuals can do for their heart health. The benefits of quitting begin almost immediately and continue to improve over time, significantly reducing the risk of heart disease and other health problems.

Obesity is another major risk factor for heart disease. Excess body weight, particularly around the abdomen, is associated with high blood pressure, high cholesterol, and diabetes—all of which increase the risk of heart disease. Achieving and maintaining a healthy weight through a balanced diet and regular physical activity can significantly reduce these risks. Even modest weight loss can have a positive impact on heart health.

Physical inactivity is a pervasive issue in modern society, with sedentary lifestyles becoming increasingly common. Regular physical activity strengthens the heart muscle, improves blood circulation, helps maintain a healthy weight, and reduces the risk of high blood pressure, high cholesterol, and diabetes. The American Heart Association recommends at least 150 minutes of moderate-intensity aerobic activity or 75 minutes of vigorous activity per week, along with muscle-strengthening activities on two or more days a week.

Diabetes, particularly type 2 diabetes, significantly increases the risk of heart disease. High blood sugar levels can damage blood vessels and the nerves that control the heart. Managing diabetes through lifestyle changes, such as a healthy diet, regular physical activity, maintaining a healthy weight, and, if necessary, medication, is crucial. Regular monitoring of blood sugar levels and working closely with healthcare providers can help manage diabetes and reduce the risk of heart disease.

Stress, often overlooked, can also impact heart health. Chronic stress may contribute to high blood pressure and other heart disease risk factors. Finding healthy ways to manage stress, such as through exercise, relaxation techniques, and positive social interactions, is important for maintaining heart health. Mindfulness and meditation practices have been shown to reduce stress and improve overall well-being, including heart health.

A heart-healthy diet is a cornerstone of cardiovascular health. The Mediterranean diet, rich in fruits, vegetables, whole grains, lean proteins, and healthy fats, is often recommended for its heart-protective benefits. Reducing the intake of processed foods, sugary beverages, and excessive amounts of red meat can also support heart health. Incorporating foods high in omega-3 fatty acids, such as fish, flaxseeds, and walnuts, can further benefit the heart by reducing inflammation and improving cholesterol levels.

Regular medical check-ups and screenings are vital for detecting and managing heart disease risk factors early. Blood pressure measurements, cholesterol level checks, blood sugar tests, and other assessments can identify potential issues before they become severe. Early detection and intervention can prevent many heart-related problems and improve outcomes for those with existing heart conditions.

In addition to individual actions, public health policies and community programs play an essential role in promoting heart health. Initiatives that encourage physical activity, provide access to healthy foods, reduce tobacco use, and manage chronic diseases can have a significant impact on population-level heart health. Advocacy for policies that support healthy environments, such as smoke-free laws and urban planning that promotes active transportation, is crucial for creating a heart-healthy society.

Education and awareness are key components of heart health. Understanding the importance of heart health and the steps one can take to protect it empowers individuals to make informed choices. Public health campaigns, educational programs, and healthcare provider guidance can raise awareness about heart disease risk factors and promote heart-healthy behaviors.

Common Heart Conditions

Heart conditions encompass a wide array of ailments that affect the cardiovascular system, each with unique characteristics, causes, and treatments. Understanding these conditions is crucial, as early detection and proper management can significantly improve outcomes and quality of life. Let's delve into some of the most common heart conditions, exploring their causes, symptoms, and treatment options.

Coronary artery disease (CAD) is the most prevalent heart condition, often leading to heart attacks. CAD occurs when the coronary arteries, which supply blood to the heart muscle, become narrowed or blocked due to a build-up of plaque—a mixture of fat, cholesterol, and other substances. This process, known as atherosclerosis, reduces blood flow to the heart, causing chest pain (angina) and, if a blockage occurs, a heart attack. Risk factors for CAD include high blood pressure, high cholesterol, smoking, diabetes, obesity, and a sedentary lifestyle. Treatment typically involves lifestyle changes, medications to manage risk factors, and in severe cases, surgical procedures like angioplasty or coronary artery bypass grafting (CABG).

Heart failure, sometimes referred to as congestive heart failure, is another common condition where the heart is unable to pump blood effectively. This can result from various underlying issues, including CAD, high blood pressure, and previous heart attacks that have weakened the heart muscle. Symptoms include shortness of breath, swelling in the legs and ankles, fatigue, and persistent coughing or wheezing. Management of heart failure often involves a combination of lifestyle changes, medications, and sometimes devices like pacemakers or defibrillators to help the heart function more efficiently. In advanced cases, a heart transplant may be considered.

Arrhythmias, or irregular heartbeats, can range from benign to life-threatening. The heart relies on electrical impulses to beat in a regular rhythm, and arrhythmias occur when these impulses are disrupted. Common types include atrial fibrillation (AFib), where the upper chambers of the heart (atria) beat irregularly, and ventricular tachycardia, a fast and potentially dangerous rhythm originating in the heart's lower chambers (ventricles). Symptoms can include palpitations, dizziness, shortness of breath, and chest pain. Treatment depends on the type and severity of the arrhythmia and may include medications, electrical cardioversion (a procedure to reset the heart's rhythm), catheter ablation (destroying the tissue causing the abnormal rhythm), or implantable devices like pacemakers and defibrillators.

Valvular heart disease involves damage or defects in one or more of the heart's valves, which control blood flow through the heart's chambers. The most common types are aortic stenosis (narrowing of the aortic valve) and mitral regurgitation (leakage of the mitral valve). Valvular disease can be congenital (present at birth) or acquired due to factors like aging, infections (such as rheumatic fever), or other heart conditions. Symptoms may include fatigue, shortness of breath, swelling in the legs, and chest pain. Treatment options range from medications to manage symptoms to surgical repair or replacement of the affected valve, often using minimally invasive techniques.

Cardiomyopathy refers to diseases of the heart muscle that make it harder for the heart to pump blood. There are several types, including dilated cardiomyopathy (where the heart becomes enlarged and weakened), hypertrophic cardiomyopathy (where the heart muscle thickens abnormally), and restrictive cardiomyopathy (where the heart muscle becomes rigid and less elastic). Causes can be genetic, due to other diseases, or idiopathic (unknown). Symptoms often include fatigue, shortness of breath, and swelling in the legs. Treatment focuses on managing symptoms and may involve medications, lifestyle changes, and in severe cases, devices like defibrillators or heart transplants.

Congenital heart defects are structural problems with the heart present at birth. These defects can range from simple issues like small holes in the heart's walls to complex malformations involving multiple parts of the heart. Advances in medical and surgical treatments have significantly improved the prognosis for many congenital heart defects, allowing individuals to lead full and active lives. Symptoms and treatments vary widely depending on the specific defect and its severity. Some defects may require surgical correction shortly after birth, while others may be managed with medications and regular monitoring.

Pericarditis is an inflammation of the pericardium, the sac-like membrane surrounding the heart. It can be caused by infections, autoimmune diseases, or other medical conditions. Symptoms often include sharp chest pain that may worsen with deep breathing, fever, and a feeling of weakness or fatigue. Treatment typically involves medications to reduce inflammation and manage pain. In some cases, if fluid accumulates around the heart (pericardial effusion), more invasive procedures may be necessary to drain the fluid and relieve pressure on the heart.

Myocarditis is an inflammation of the heart muscle itself, usually caused by viral infections, though it can also result from bacterial infections, autoimmune diseases, or exposure to certain toxins. Symptoms can mimic those of other heart conditions, such as chest pain, fatigue, shortness of breath, and arrhythmias. Diagnosing myocarditis often requires blood tests, imaging studies, and sometimes a biopsy of the heart tissue. Treatment focuses on addressing the underlying cause and managing symptoms, which may include medications to reduce inflammation and support heart function.

Heart attacks, or myocardial infarctions, occur when blood flow to a part of the heart is blocked, usually by a blood clot, leading to damage or death of heart muscle tissue. Immediate symptoms include intense chest pain, shortness of breath, nausea, and lightheadedness. Prompt medical treatment is crucial to restore blood flow and minimize heart damage. Treatment typically involves medications to dissolve clots or prevent further clotting, as well as procedures like angioplasty to open blocked arteries and restore blood flow.

Preventing and managing heart conditions often involves a combination of lifestyle changes, medications, and regular medical care. A heart-healthy lifestyle includes a balanced diet rich in fruits, vegetables, whole grains, and lean proteins, regular physical activity, maintaining a healthy weight, avoiding tobacco, and limiting alcohol consumption. Regular check-ups with healthcare providers are essential for monitoring heart health and managing risk factors like high blood pressure, high cholesterol, and diabetes.

Medications play a crucial role in the management of many heart conditions. These can include antihypertensives to control high blood pressure, statins to lower cholesterol, anticoagulants to prevent blood clots, and various other drugs tailored to specific conditions. It is important for individuals to work closely with their healthcare providers to ensure that their medication regimens are effective and to adjust them as needed based on their evolving health status.

Surgical and procedural interventions are often necessary for more serious heart conditions. Advances in medical technology have led to the development of minimally invasive techniques that can reduce recovery times and improve outcomes for patients. These include procedures like angioplasty, stenting, and minimally invasive valve repair or replacement. In some cases, more invasive surgeries such as coronary artery bypass grafting (CABG) or heart transplantation may be required.

Overview of Cardiac Treatments

Cardiac treatments have evolved significantly over the past few decades, offering a range of options tailored to the specific needs of individuals with heart disease. From lifestyle modifications and medications to advanced surgical procedures, understanding the array of treatments available is crucial for managing heart conditions effectively.

Lifestyle changes are often the first line of defense in treating heart disease. Adopting a heart-healthy diet is paramount. This typically includes increasing the intake of fruits, vegetables, whole grains, and lean proteins while reducing saturated fats, trans fats, cholesterol, and sodium. For example, the

Mediterranean diet, rich in olive oil, fish, and nuts, has been shown to reduce the risk of heart disease. Regular physical activity is equally important. The American Heart Association recommends at least 150 minutes of moderate-intensity aerobic exercise or 75 minutes of vigorous exercise each week, supplemented by muscle-strengthening activities. Quitting smoking is another critical step, as tobacco use is a major risk factor for cardiovascular diseases. Similarly, managing stress through mindfulness, meditation, or other relaxation techniques can have a positive impact on heart health.

Medications play a pivotal role in the management of heart disease. There are several classes of drugs that healthcare providers commonly prescribe. Antihypertensives, such as ACE inhibitors, beta-blockers, and calcium channel blockers, help control high blood pressure, a major risk factor for heart disease. Statins and other lipid-lowering agents are used to manage high cholesterol levels. Anticoagulants and antiplatelet drugs, like aspirin and warfarin, are prescribed to prevent blood clots that can lead to heart attacks and strokes. Diuretics help reduce fluid build-up in the body, easing the workload on the heart, particularly in patients with heart failure. It is crucial for patients to adhere to their medication regimens and to communicate regularly with their healthcare providers to adjust dosages as necessary and to manage any side effects that may arise.

For some individuals, lifestyle changes and medications may not be sufficient, and more invasive treatments may be required. One common procedure is angioplasty, often accompanied by the placement of a stent. During angioplasty, a catheter with a balloon at its tip is inserted into a narrowed artery. The balloon is then inflated to widen the artery, and a stent—a small wire mesh tube—is placed to keep the artery open. This procedure can significantly improve blood flow and reduce symptoms such as chest pain. In more severe cases of coronary artery disease, coronary artery bypass grafting (CABG) may be necessary. This surgery involves taking a healthy blood vessel from another part of the body and using it to bypass a blocked coronary artery, thereby restoring adequate blood flow to the heart muscle.

Arrhythmias, or irregular heartbeats, often require specialized treatments. For instance, atrial fibrillation (AFib), a common type of arrhythmia, can be managed with medications that control the heart rate or rhythm. In some cases, electrical cardioversion may be performed to restore a normal heart rhythm. Another option is catheter ablation, a procedure in which a catheter is used to destroy small areas of heart tissue that are causing the abnormal rhythm.

For more serious arrhythmias, implantable devices such as pacemakers and defibrillators may be necessary. Pacemakers help regulate the heartbeat, while implantable cardioverter-defibrillators (ICDs) can detect and correct life-threatening arrhythmias by delivering an electric shock to the heart.

Valvular heart diseases, such as aortic stenosis or mitral regurgitation, often require surgical intervention. Traditional open-heart surgery to repair or replace a damaged valve is one option. However, less invasive techniques have become increasingly popular. For example, transcatheter aortic valve replacement (TAVR) allows a new valve to be inserted via a catheter, avoiding the need for open-heart surgery. Similarly, mitral valve repair can sometimes be performed using minimally invasive techniques, reducing recovery times and improving outcomes for patients.

Heart failure, a condition in which the heart cannot pump enough blood to meet the body's needs, often requires a multifaceted treatment approach. In addition to lifestyle changes and medications, certain devices can help manage the condition. Cardiac resynchronization therapy (CRT), for instance, uses a special type of pacemaker to improve the timing of the heart's contractions, enhancing its ability to pump blood. For patients with severe heart failure, a left ventricular assist device (LVAD) may be implanted to help the heart pump blood. In the most extreme cases, a heart transplant may be considered. Advances in immunosuppressive therapies have improved the success rates of transplants, allowing many recipients to enjoy a good quality of life post-surgery.

For congenital heart defects, which are structural problems present at birth, treatment varies widely depending on the specific defect and its severity. Some defects may close on their own and require only monitoring, while others might necessitate surgical correction soon after birth. Advances in pediatric cardiology have significantly improved the outcomes for children with congenital heart defects, enabling many to lead healthy, active lives. Procedures such as the repair of atrial or ventricular septal defects (holes in the heart's walls) or complex surgeries for conditions like Tetralogy of Fallot have become routine in specialized centers.

In addition to these physical treatments, psychological support and rehabilitation are crucial components of comprehensive cardiac care. Cardiac rehabilitation programs, which combine supervised exercise, education, and counseling, can help patients recover after a heart attack, surgery, or other heart events. These programs aim to improve cardiovascular fitness, reduce risk factors, and help patients adopt a heart-healthy lifestyle. Emotional support, whether through counseling, support groups, or therapy, is equally important, as heart disease can take a significant toll on mental health. Addressing anxiety, depression, and other psychological issues can improve overall well-being and enhance recovery.

Innovations in cardiac treatment continue to emerge, driven by ongoing research and technological advancements. For example, regenerative medicine, including stem cell therapy, holds promise for repairing damaged heart tissue and improving heart function. Similarly, advances in imaging techniques, such as cardiac MRI and CT scans, allow for more precise diagnosis and treatment planning. Personalized medicine, which tailors treatment based on an individual's genetic makeup, is another exciting frontier in cardiology, potentially leading to more effective and targeted therapies.

Chapter 2

Anatomy and Physiology of the Heart

Structure of the Heart

The human heart, a marvel of biological engineering, is a muscular organ about the size of a fist. It functions as the central component of the circulatory system, tirelessly pumping blood throughout the body to supply oxygen and nutrients while removing waste products. Understanding the intricate structure of the heart is essential for appreciating its role in health and disease.

The heart is divided into four chambers: two atria and two ventricles. The atria are the upper chambers, and their primary function is to receive blood returning to the heart from the body and lungs. The right atrium receives deoxygenated blood from the superior and inferior vena cava, which are large veins that collect blood from the body. The left atrium receives oxygenated blood from the lungs through the pulmonary veins. The atria are separated from the ventricles by valves that prevent backflow of blood, ensuring unidirectional flow.

The ventricles, the lower chambers of the heart, are responsible for pumping blood out of the heart. The right ventricle pumps deoxygenated blood into the pulmonary artery, which carries it to the lungs for oxygenation. The left ventricle, the most muscular and powerful chamber, pumps oxygenated blood into the aorta, the largest artery in the body, which distributes it to the systemic circulation. The robust structure of the left ventricle is necessary to generate the high pressure required to deliver blood throughout the entire body.

The heart's anatomy includes four key valves: the tricuspid valve, the pulmonary valve, the mitral valve, and the aortic valve. The tricuspid valve, located between the right atrium and right ventricle, has three leaflets that open to allow blood flow into the right ventricle and close to prevent backflow. The pulmonary valve is situated between the right ventricle and the pulmonary artery. It opens to permit blood flow into the lungs and closes to prevent it from flowing back into the right ventricle. On the left side of the heart, the mitral valve, also known as the bicuspid valve due to its two leaflets, controls blood flow between the left atrium and left ventricle. The aortic valve is positioned between the left ventricle and the aorta, opening to allow blood to enter the systemic circulation and closing to prevent backflow into the left ventricle.

The heart's walls are composed of three layers: the endocardium, myocardium, and epicardium. The endocardium is the innermost layer, a thin, smooth membrane that lines the interior of the heart chambers and valves, providing a frictionless surface for blood flow. The myocardium, the thick middle layer, is composed of cardiac muscle tissue. This layer is responsible for the heart's contractile function, enabling it to pump blood. The outermost layer, the epicardium, is a thin layer of connective tissue that serves as a protective covering. It is continuous with the visceral layer of the pericardium, a double-walled sac that encases the heart, providing additional protection and reducing friction during heartbeats.

The heart's electrical conduction system is fundamental to its ability to function as an effective pump. The sinoatrial (SA) node, located in the right atrium, is often referred to as the natural pacemaker of the heart. It generates electrical impulses that spread across the atria, causing them to contract and push blood into the ventricles. The atrioventricular (AV) node, situated at the junction between the atria and ventricles, acts as a gatekeeper, momentarily delaying the electrical signal to ensure the atria have emptied their blood into the ventricles before they contract. From the AV node, the impulse travels through the bundle of His, which divides into right and left bundle branches along the interventricular septum, and then into the Purkinje fibers that extend throughout the ventricular myocardium, causing the ventricles to contract and eject blood either to the lungs or the systemic circulation.

The coronary arteries play a vital role in supplying the heart muscle with oxygenated blood. The two primary coronary arteries, the left and right coronary arteries, originate from the base of the aorta. The left coronary artery further branches into the left anterior descending artery and the circumflex artery, which supply the front and left side of the heart. The right coronary artery supplies the right side of the heart and usually gives rise to the posterior descending artery, which supplies the back of the heart. Adequate blood flow through these arteries is crucial for maintaining the myocardial function and health.

In addition to its structural components, the heart operates within a complex regulatory framework influenced by neural and hormonal factors. The autonomic nervous system, comprising the sympathetic and parasympathetic nervous systems, plays a significant role in heart rate and contractility regulation. The sympathetic nervous system increases heart rate and the force of contraction during stress or physical activity, while the parasympathetic nervous system slows the heart rate during rest. Hormones such as adrenaline and noradrenaline, released by the adrenal glands, also enhance heart rate and contractility during times of stress.

The heart's structure and function are closely intertwined, and any disruption in one can significantly affect the other. For instance, coronary artery disease results from the buildup of plaques in the coronary arteries, reducing blood flow to the myocardium and potentially leading to heart attacks. Similarly, valvular heart diseases, such as stenosis (narrowing of the valves) or regurgitation (leakage of the valves), can impair the heart's ability to pump blood effectively, leading to heart failure if untreated.

Congenital heart defects, structural abnormalities present at birth, can also impact heart function. These defects may involve the septum, valves, or major arteries and veins associated with the heart. Some common congenital defects include atrial septal defects (holes in the wall between the atria), ventricular septal defects (holes in the wall between the ventricles), and Tetralogy of Fallot, which involves four anatomical abnormalities leading to reduced oxygenation of blood.

Blood Circulation Pathways

Blood circulation pathways are the lifelines of the human body, ensuring that every cell receives the oxygen and nutrients it needs while removing waste products. The circulatory system is a closed network of vessels that includes the heart, arteries, veins, and capillaries, all working together to maintain the continuous flow of blood. This system can be divided into two main circuits: the pulmonary circulation and the systemic circulation, each with distinct roles but interconnected functions.

Pulmonary circulation begins in the right ventricle of the heart. When the heart contracts, it sends deoxygenated blood into the pulmonary artery, the only artery in the body that carries oxygen-poor blood. This artery branches into smaller arteries, arterioles, and finally into the capillary networks within the lungs. Here, blood undergoes a critical transformation. As blood flows through the lung capillaries, it releases carbon dioxide, a waste product of cellular metabolism, and absorbs oxygen from the air we breathe. This gas exchange is facilitated by the thin walls of the alveoli, the tiny air sacs in the lungs. Oxygenated blood then travels through the pulmonary veins, the only veins that carry oxygen-rich blood, back to the left atrium of the heart. From here, it moves into the left ventricle, ready to be pumped into the systemic circulation.

Systemic circulation is the pathway that delivers oxygenated blood from the heart to the rest of the body and returns deoxygenated blood back to the heart. This journey starts when the left ventricle contracts, sending blood into the aorta, the largest artery in the body. The aorta arches and extends downward, giving rise to major arteries that supply blood to the head, arms, and lower body. As arteries branch into smaller arterioles and capillaries, they reach every tissue and organ. Capillaries, with their thin walls, are the sites of nutrient and gas exchange. Oxygen and nutrients diffuse from the blood into the tissues, while carbon dioxide and metabolic wastes move from the tissues into the blood.

After the exchange in the capillaries, blood begins its return journey to the heart. Capillaries merge into venules, which in turn merge into larger veins. Blood from the upper body is collected by the superior vena cava, while blood from the lower body is collected by the inferior vena cava. Both vena cavae empty into the right atrium of the heart, completing the systemic circuit. From the right atrium, blood moves into the right ventricle, ready to be sent back to the lungs via pulmonary circulation.

Beyond these primary circuits, the circulatory system includes specialized pathways that serve specific functions. The coronary circulation, for example, is the network of vessels that supply blood to the heart muscle itself. The heart, like any other tissue, requires a constant supply of oxygen and nutrients to function. The coronary arteries branch off from the base of the aorta and encircle the heart, penetrating the myocardium to deliver oxygen-rich blood. After the oxygen is used, deoxygenated blood is collected by the coronary veins, which drain into the right atrium through the coronary sinus.

Another specialized pathway is the hepatic portal circulation, which carries nutrient-rich blood from the digestive organs to the liver. After a meal, blood leaving the stomach and intestines is laden with absorbed nutrients. Instead of going directly back to the heart, this blood is diverted to the liver via the hepatic portal vein. In the liver, nutrients are processed, stored, or detoxified before the blood continues its journey to the heart. This system allows the liver to regulate blood nutrient levels and detoxify substances absorbed from the intestines.

The brain also has a unique circulatory pathway known as the cerebral circulation. The brain consumes a significant portion of the body's oxygen and glucose, making consistent blood flow critical. Blood reaches the brain through the carotid arteries and vertebral arteries, which join to form the Circle of Willis, a ring-like arterial structure that provides multiple pathways for blood to reach the brain. This redundancy ensures that if one route is blocked, others can compensate, protecting the brain from ischemia.

The lymphatic system, though not part of the cardiovascular system, works in parallel with it. It helps maintain fluid balance by returning excess interstitial fluid to the bloodstream and plays a role in immune defense. Lymphatic vessels collect interstitial fluid, now called lymph, and transport it through lymph nodes where it is filtered. The lymphatic system eventually empties into the subclavian veins, returning the filtered fluid to the circulatory system.

Understanding blood circulation pathways is crucial for recognizing how the body maintains homeostasis and responds to various challenges. For instance, during physical activity, the body adjusts blood flow to meet the increased oxygen and nutrient demands of muscles. The heart rate and stroke volume increase, and blood vessels in muscles dilate to enhance blood flow. Conversely, blood flow to non-essential areas like the digestive system may decrease temporarily to prioritize muscle perfusion.

In pathological conditions, circulation can be severely affected. Atherosclerosis, the buildup of plaques in arteries, can lead to reduced blood flow and increased risk of heart attack or stroke. Hypertension, or high blood pressure, forces the heart to work harder and can damage blood vessels over time. Varicose veins occur when veins become enlarged and overfilled with blood, often due to faulty valves that fail to maintain unidirectional blood flow.

Medical interventions often aim to restore or enhance circulation. Procedures such as angioplasty or coronary artery bypass grafting (CABG) are used to treat blocked coronary arteries. Medications like anticoagulants or antihypertensives manage conditions that affect blood flow. Lifestyle changes, including diet and exercise, play a significant role in maintaining healthy circulation.

Electrical System of the Heart

The heart's ability to pump blood efficiently throughout the body hinges on a precisely coordinated electrical system. This system initiates and regulates the heart's rhythmic contractions, ensuring that blood is propelled in a timely and organized manner. The heartbeat, a seemingly simple phenomenon, is the result of a complex interplay between various electrical components within the heart. Understanding this electrical system is crucial for comprehending how the heart functions normally and what happens when it malfunctions.

The journey of an electrical impulse in the heart begins in the sinoatrial (SA) node, often referred to as the heart's natural pacemaker. Located in the right atrium near the opening of the superior vena cava, the SA node generates electrical impulses at regular intervals. These impulses are spontaneous, arising from the unique properties of the pacemaker cells, which possess a natural ability to depolarize without any external stimulus. The rate at which these impulses are generated dictates the heart rate, typically ranging from 60 to 100 beats per minute in a healthy adult at rest.

Once generated, the electrical impulse quickly spreads across the atria, causing the atrial muscle cells to depolarize and contract. This contraction propels blood from the atria into the ventricles. The movement of the impulse through the atria is facilitated by specialized pathways, including Bachmann's bundle, which ensures synchronized contraction of both atria. This coordinated atrial contraction is essential for optimizing ventricular filling and maintaining efficient cardiac output.

After traversing the atria, the electrical impulse reaches the atrioventricular (AV) node, situated at the junction between the atria and ventricles. The AV node serves as a critical gatekeeper, introducing a deliberate delay in the transmission of the impulse to the ventricles. This delay, lasting approximately 0.1 seconds, allows the ventricles sufficient time to fill with blood before they contract. Without this delay, the ventricles would contract too early, reducing their efficiency in pumping blood.

From the AV node, the impulse travels along the bundle of His, a specialized pathway that penetrates the interventricular septum. The bundle of His quickly bifurcates into the right and left bundle branches, which extend down either side of the septum toward the apex of the heart. These branches are crucial for directing the electrical impulse to the appropriate regions of the ventricles, ensuring a coordinated and effective contraction.

The terminal part of the electrical conduction system involves the Purkinje fibers, a network of fibers that spread throughout the ventricular myocardium. The Purkinje fibers conduct the electrical impulse at a rapid pace, allowing for a swift and uniform depolarization of the ventricular muscle cells. This rapid conduction is vital for producing a strong and coordinated ventricular contraction, propelling blood into the pulmonary artery from the right ventricle and into the aorta from the left ventricle.

The entire sequence of electrical events, from the SA node to the Purkinje fibers, occurs within a fraction of a second, resulting in the synchronized and rhythmic contraction of the heart. This process is meticulously regulated by the intrinsic properties of the heart's electrical cells and the autonomic nervous system. The sympathetic nervous system can increase the heart rate and force of contraction during periods of stress or physical activity, while the parasympathetic nervous system can slow the heart rate during restful periods.

Disturbances in the heart's electrical system can lead to arrhythmias, conditions characterized by abnormal heart rhythms. Arrhythmias can range from benign to life-threatening, depending on their nature and origin. Tachycardia, a condition where the heart beats faster than normal, can arise from increased automaticity of the SA node, atrial fibrillation, or ventricular tachycardia. Conversely, bradycardia, a slower than normal heart rate, may result from SA node dysfunction or AV block, where the transmission of impulses through the AV node is impaired.

Atrial fibrillation, one of the most common arrhythmias, involves rapid and irregular electrical impulses in the atria, leading to ineffective atrial contractions. This can result in incomplete ventricular filling and a reduction in cardiac output. Additionally, the irregular rhythm increases the risk of blood clot formation in the atria, which can travel to the brain and cause a stroke. Treatment for atrial fibrillation may include medications to control the heart rate and rhythm, anticoagulants to prevent clot formation, and procedures such as electrical cardioversion or catheter ablation to restore normal rhythm.

Ventricular tachycardia and ventricular fibrillation are particularly dangerous arrhythmias originating in the ventricles. Ventricular tachycardia involves a rapid heart rate arising from abnormal electrical activity within the ventricles, which can compromise cardiac output and lead to hemodynamic instability. Ventricular fibrillation, characterized by chaotic and ineffective electrical activity in the ventricles, results in the cessation of effective blood pumping and requires immediate medical intervention, typically in the form of defibrillation, to restore a normal rhythm.

To diagnose and manage arrhythmias, healthcare providers rely on tools such as the electrocardiogram (ECG or EKG). An ECG records the electrical activity of the heart through electrodes placed on the skin, providing valuable information about the heart's rhythm and identifying abnormalities in the conduction system. For instance, the P wave on an ECG represents atrial depolarization, the QRS complex corresponds to ventricular depolarization, and the T wave reflects ventricular repolarization. By analyzing these waveforms and intervals, clinicians can pinpoint the location and nature of electrical disturbances.

In addition to the ECG, advanced diagnostic tools and techniques such as Holter monitoring, event recorders, and electrophysiological studies can provide further insights into the heart's electrical activity. Holter monitors are portable devices worn by patients to continuously record heart activity over 24 to 48 hours, capturing arrhythmias that may not occur during a standard ECG. Electrophysiological studies involve inserting catheters into the heart to directly measure electrical activity and identify abnormal pathways, often guiding therapeutic interventions like catheter ablation.

Treatment for arrhythmias may include medications that modify the electrical properties of the heart cells, such as beta-blockers, calcium channel blockers, antiarrhythmics, and lifestyle modifications to reduce triggers of abnormal rhythms. Catheter ablation is a minimally invasive procedure used to destroy small areas of heart tissue that give rise to abnormal electrical signals, effectively curing certain types of arrhythmias. In more severe cases, implantable devices such as pacemakers and implantable cardioverter-defibrillators (ICDs) may be necessary. Pacemakers help regulate a slow heart rate by delivering electrical impulses to stimulate heartbeats, while ICDs monitor the heart's rhythm and deliver shocks to terminate life-threatening arrhythmias.

Cardiac Cycle and Heart Sounds

The heart's ability to pump blood effectively throughout the body hinges on the intricate sequence of events known as the cardiac cycle. This cycle encompasses the periods of contraction and relaxation of the heart chambers, ensuring the efficient movement of blood. Each phase of the cardiac cycle corresponds to specific heart sounds, offering vital clues about the heart's function and potential abnormalities. Understanding the cardiac cycle and the associated heart sounds is fundamental for anyone delving into cardiovascular health and diagnostics.

The cardiac cycle begins with atrial systole, the phase where the atria contract to push blood into the ventricles. This phase is preceded by the passive filling of the ventricles during diastole. As the atria contract, the pressure within them increases, forcing the atrioventricular (AV) valves—comprising the mitral valve on the left side and the tricuspid valve on the right—to open wider, allowing blood to flow into the ventricles. This phase, though brief, is crucial as it ensures the ventricles receive an adequate volume of blood to pump out during the next contraction.

As atrial systole ends, ventricular systole begins. During this phase, the ventricles contract, generating pressure that closes the AV valves, preventing backflow into the atria. The closure of these valves produces the first heart sound, known as "S1" or "lub." This sound signifies the onset of ventricular contraction and is a key indicator of the heart's mechanical activity. The pressure within the ventricles continues to rise until it exceeds the pressure in the aorta and pulmonary artery, prompting the opening of the semilunar valves—the aortic valve on the left and the pulmonary valve on the right.

Blood is then ejected from the ventricles into the systemic and pulmonary circulation. This ejection phase is marked by a rapid outflow of blood, followed by a slower phase as the pressure gradients equalize. Efficient ejection ensures that sufficient blood reaches the organs and tissues to meet metabolic demands. Any disruption in this phase, such as in conditions like aortic stenosis, can significantly impact the body's oxygenation and nutrient supply.

Following the ejection phase, the ventricles begin to relax, entering the period known as ventricular diastole. As the ventricular pressure falls below the pressure in the aorta and pulmonary artery, the semilunar valves close, producing the second heart sound, "S2" or "dub." This sound marks the end of systole and the beginning of diastole. The closure of the semilunar valves prevents the backflow of blood into the ventricles, a critical aspect of maintaining unidirectional blood flow.

Diastole is characterized by the relaxation and filling of the ventricles. During this phase, the ventricles expand, and the pressure within them drops, allowing the AV valves to open once again. Blood flows passively from the atria into the ventricles, facilitated by the pressure gradient. This period of passive filling is essential for ensuring that the ventricles are adequately filled without the need for atrial contraction. The cycle then repeats with the next atrial systole.

Heart sounds provide a wealth of information about the cardiac cycle and can reveal underlying pathologies. The first and second heart sounds, S1 and S2, are the most prominent and are typically heard during a routine physical examination. However, additional heart sounds, such as the third heart sound (S3) and the fourth heart sound (S4), can also be present and may indicate specific cardiac conditions.

The third heart sound, S3, occurs during the rapid filling phase of diastole. It is often heard in young, healthy individuals and athletes, where it is considered a normal variant. However, in older adults or those with heart disease, an S3 can indicate increased ventricular filling pressures, often seen in conditions such as heart failure or dilated cardiomyopathy. The presence of an S3 warrants further investigation to determine the underlying cause and appropriate management.

The fourth heart sound, S4, occurs just before S1, during atrial systole. It is produced by the atria contracting against a stiff or non-compliant ventricle. S4 is often associated with conditions that cause ventricular hypertrophy or fibrosis, such as hypertension, aortic stenosis, or ischemic heart disease. The detection of an S4 can provide critical insights into the structural and functional state of the ventricles.

Murmurs are additional sounds that can be heard during the cardiac cycle and are indicative of turbulent blood flow within the heart or great vessels. They can result from a variety of causes, including valvular stenosis, regurgitation, or congenital heart defects. The timing, location, and quality of a murmur provide valuable clues to its etiology. For instance, a systolic murmur heard best at the right sternal border often suggests aortic stenosis, whereas a diastolic murmur at the apex may indicate mitral stenosis.

The auscultation of heart sounds and murmurs is a skill that requires practice and a thorough understanding of the cardiac cycle. It involves using a stethoscope to listen to the sounds produced by the heart and interpreting them in the context of the patient's clinical presentation. Experienced clinicians can diagnose a wide range of cardiac conditions based on the nuances of these sounds, making auscultation an indispensable tool in cardiovascular assessment.

Technological advancements have complemented traditional auscultation techniques. Echocardiography, for instance, uses ultrasound waves to create detailed images of the heart's structures and motion. It can visualize valvular abnormalities, measure ventricular function, and detect the presence of fluid around the heart. Doppler echocardiography, in particular, provides information about blood flow patterns and can quantify the severity of valvular stenosis or regurgitation.

While technology enhances diagnostic capabilities, the fundamental understanding of the cardiac cycle and heart sounds remains critical. It forms the foundation upon which more advanced diagnostic modalities build. Moreover, it enables healthcare providers to make rapid, bedside assessments that can guide immediate clinical decisions.

In clinical practice, integrating knowledge of the cardiac cycle with the interpretation of heart sounds can lead to early detection of cardiac conditions. For example, recognizing the characteristic murmur of mitral regurgitation can prompt further evaluation and timely intervention, potentially preventing the progression to heart failure. Similarly, identifying the signs of aortic stenosis through auscultation can lead to early surgical consultation, improving patient outcomes.

Heart's Role in the Body

The heart, a marvel of biological engineering, serves as the centerpiece of the body's circulatory system, tirelessly pumping blood to sustain the myriad functions essential to life. Its role extends beyond merely acting as a pump; it orchestrates a complex network of vessels that deliver oxygen, nutrients, and hormones to tissues while simultaneously removing waste products. Understanding the heart's integral role in the body requires an appreciation of its structure, function, and the way it interacts with other organ systems.

At the core of the cardiovascular system, the heart is a muscular organ divided into four chambers: two atria and two ventricles. These chambers work in a coordinated manner to ensure unidirectional blood flow. The right atrium receives deoxygenated blood from the body's systemic circulation via the superior and inferior vena cava. This blood then moves into the right ventricle, which pumps it to the lungs through the pulmonary artery for oxygenation.

Oxygen-rich blood returns to the left atrium via the pulmonary veins, flows into the left ventricle, and is then ejected into the aorta, the body's main artery, to supply the systemic circulation.

The heart's ability to maintain this cycle is governed by its electrical conduction system, which ensures that the contractions of the atria and ventricles are synchronized. The sinoatrial (SA) node, often referred to as the heart's natural pacemaker, initiates the electrical impulse that triggers atrial contraction. This impulse travels to the atrioventricular (AV) node, where it is momentarily delayed to allow complete ventricular filling. The signal then proceeds through the bundle of His, branching into the right and left bundle branches, and finally disperses through the Purkinje fibers to prompt ventricular contraction. This precise timing is crucial for efficient blood circulation.

The heart's role in the body extends to its influence on blood pressure regulation, a vital aspect of homeostasis. Blood pressure, the force exerted by circulating blood on the walls of blood vessels, is tightly regulated by the heart and the vascular system. The cardiac output, defined as the volume of blood the heart pumps per minute, and the total peripheral resistance, the resistance blood encounters as it flows through the vascular system, are the primary determinants of blood pressure. The heart adjusts its output in response to the body's needs, such as during exercise or stress, ensuring adequate perfusion of tissues.

Moreover, the heart interacts with various hormones and signaling molecules that modulate cardiovascular function. For instance, the renin-angiotensin-aldosterone system (RAAS) plays a critical role in blood pressure regulation and fluid balance. When blood pressure drops, the kidneys release renin, which catalyzes the production of angiotensin II, a potent vasoconstrictor that raises blood pressure. Angiotensin II also stimulates the release of aldosterone from the adrenal glands, promoting sodium and water retention by the kidneys, thereby increasing blood volume and pressure. The heart itself secretes natriuretic peptides, such as atrial natriuretic peptide (ANP), which counteract the effects of the RAAS by promoting vasodilation and reducing blood volume.

The heart's function is also intimately linked with the respiratory system. The pulmonary circulation, managed by the right side of the heart, ensures that blood is oxygenated in the lungs. Any disruption in this process, such as in pulmonary hypertension or chronic obstructive pulmonary disease (COPD), places additional strain on the right ventricle, potentially leading to right-sided heart failure. Conversely, conditions affecting the left side of the heart, like left ventricular hypertrophy or mitral valve disease, can cause pulmonary congestion and compromise respiratory function.

Exercise physiology provides a clear illustration of the heart's adaptability and its broader role in maintaining bodily function. During physical activity, the demand for oxygen and nutrients in muscles increases significantly. The heart meets this demand by increasing both the heart rate (chronotropy) and the force of contractions (inotropy), thereby boosting cardiac output. The enhanced blood flow delivers more oxygen to active muscles and facilitates the removal of metabolic byproducts like carbon dioxide and lactic acid. Regular exercise strengthens the heart muscle, improves its efficiency, and enhances the overall cardiovascular health, reducing the risk of heart disease.

The heart's role is not confined to the circulatory and respiratory systems; it also impacts other organ systems. For instance, the kidneys rely on consistent blood flow to filter waste products from the blood and maintain fluid and electrolyte balance. Any compromise in cardiac function, such as in heart failure, can lead to reduced renal perfusion, impairing kidney function and exacerbating fluid retention, which further burdens the heart. Additionally, the gastrointestinal system depends on adequate blood supply for nutrient absorption and digestion. Conditions like mesenteric ischemia, where blood flow to the intestines is reduced, can have severe consequences, highlighting the heart's critical role in sustaining digestive health.

Emotional and psychological well-being are also influenced by heart health. The heart-brain connection, mediated through the autonomic nervous system, plays a significant role in stress responses. The sympathetic nervous system, which governs the "fight or flight" response, increases heart rate and contractility during stress, preparing the body for immediate action. Chronic stress, however, can lead to sustained elevated heart rates and blood pressure, increasing the risk of cardiovascular diseases. Techniques like mindfulness, meditation, and regular physical activity can mitigate these effects by promoting parasympathetic (rest and digest) activity, which calms the heart and reduces stress levels.

In the realm of medical diagnostics, the heart's role is illuminated through various investigative tools. Electrocardiography (ECG) measures the electrical activity of the heart, providing insights into its rhythm and identifying abnormalities like arrhythmias or myocardial infarction. Echocardiography uses ultrasound waves to visualize heart structures and assess function, revealing conditions such as valvular defects, congenital anomalies, or cardiomyopathies. These diagnostic modalities underscore the importance of the heart in overall health and the need for vigilant monitoring to detect and address cardiovascular issues early.

Preventive cardiology emphasizes the importance of lifestyle choices in maintaining heart health. Diet, exercise, and stress management are cornerstones of cardiovascular prevention. A diet rich in fruits, vegetables, whole grains, and lean proteins supports heart health by providing essential nutrients and minimizing risk factors like hypertension and hyperlipidemia. Regular physical activity, as previously discussed, strengthens the heart and improves vascular function. Managing stress through techniques like yoga, deep breathing exercises, or hobbies can reduce the negative impact of chronic stress on the heart.

Chapter 3

Risk Factors for Heart Disease

Genetic Factors

Genetic factors play a pivotal role in shaping an individual's health, influencing everything from susceptibility to diseases to physical traits like height and eye color. The study of genetics delves into how traits are inherited from one generation to the next through genes, which are segments of DNA located on chromosomes. Each person inherits a unique combination of genes from their parents, contributing to their genetic makeup or genotype. This chapter explores the intricate ways in which genetic factors impact health and the mechanisms by which genetic information is transferred and expressed.

At the core of genetics lies the DNA molecule, a double-helix structure composed of nucleotide pairs. These nucleotides are adenine (A), thymine (T), cytosine (C), and guanine (G), which pair specifically (A with T, and C with G) to form the rungs of the DNA ladder. The sequence of these nucleotides encodes the genetic instructions necessary for the development, functioning, and reproduction of living organisms. Genes, which are specific sequences of these nucleotides, act as blueprints for the synthesis of proteins, the workhorses of the cell that perform a vast array of functions.

The transmission of genetic information from parents to offspring occurs through the process of reproduction. Humans have 23 pairs of chromosomes, with one chromosome of each pair inherited from each parent. This means that individuals receive half of their genetic material from their mother and half from their father. During the formation of gametes (sperm and egg cells), a type of cell division called meiosis ensures that each gamete contains only one set of chromosomes. When fertilization occurs, the union of sperm and egg restores the diploid state, with the resulting zygote containing a full set of chromosomes.

Genetic variation among individuals arises through several mechanisms, including mutations, genetic recombination, and the independent assortment of chromosomes during meiosis. Mutations are changes in the DNA sequence that can occur spontaneously or due to environmental factors such as radiation or chemicals. While many mutations are neutral or harmful, some can confer advantageous traits that enhance survival and reproduction. Genetic recombination, which occurs during meiosis, involves the exchange of genetic material between homologous chromosomes, creating new combinations of alleles. This shuffling of genetic information contributes to the diversity observed within populations.

Certain genetic factors are associated with an increased risk of developing specific diseases. For example, mutations in the BRCA1 and BRCA2 genes significantly elevate the risk of breast and ovarian cancers. Individuals who inherit these mutations may undergo more frequent screenings and consider preventive measures to reduce their risk. Similarly, the presence of the APOE ε4 allele is linked to a higher likelihood of developing Alzheimer's disease. Understanding these genetic risk factors can lead to personalized medicine approaches, where prevention and treatment strategies are tailored to an individual's genetic profile.

One of the most well-known examples of genetic inheritance is Mendelian inheritance, named after Gregor Mendel, the father of genetics. Mendel's experiments with pea plants in the 19th century revealed that traits are inherited in predictable patterns through dominant and recessive alleles. For instance, a child must inherit two copies of the recessive allele for cystic fibrosis (one from each parent) to manifest the disease. If they inherit only one copy, they will be a carrier but will not exhibit symptoms. These principles of inheritance apply to many other genetic conditions, such as sickle cell anemia and Tay-Sachs disease.

However, not all genetic traits follow simple Mendelian patterns. Many traits and diseases are influenced by multiple genes, as well as environmental factors, in what is known as multifactorial inheritance. Conditions like heart disease, diabetes, and certain types of cancer fall into this category. For instance, while genes may predispose an individual to diabetes, lifestyle factors such as diet, exercise, and weight management play crucial roles in determining whether the disease will develop. This interplay between genes and environment underscores the complexity of genetic influences on health.

Advances in genetic research have led to the identification of genetic markers associated with various diseases. Genome-wide association studies (GWAS) scan the genomes of large populations to find genetic variations linked to specific conditions. These studies have uncovered numerous genetic variants that contribute to complex diseases, providing insights into their underlying biological mechanisms. For example, GWAS have identified multiple loci associated with increased risk of type 2 diabetes, highlighting the role of genes involved in insulin secretion and glucose metabolism.

The advent of genetic testing has revolutionized the ability to diagnose and predict genetic disorders. Techniques such as polymerase chain reaction (PCR), DNA sequencing, and microarray analysis allow for the detection of genetic mutations and variations. Genetic testing can be performed prenatally, in newborns, or later in life to identify carriers of genetic conditions, diagnose diseases, or assess disease risk. For instance, newborn screening programs test for inherited metabolic disorders, enabling early intervention and treatment that can prevent severe health problems.

Ethical considerations arise in the context of genetic testing and the use of genetic information. Issues such as privacy, informed consent, and potential discrimination must be carefully addressed. The Genetic Information Nondiscrimination Act (GINA) in the United States, for example, protects individuals from discrimination based on their genetic information in health insurance and employment. Additionally, genetic counseling plays a crucial role in helping individuals understand the implications of genetic testing, interpret results, and make informed decisions about their health and reproductive choices.

Gene therapy represents a promising frontier in the treatment of genetic disorders. This approach involves introducing, removing, or altering genetic material within a person's cells to treat or prevent disease. For example, gene therapy has shown success in treating certain forms of inherited blindness and immunodeficiency disorders. By addressing the root cause of genetic diseases at the molecular level, gene therapy holds the potential to provide long-lasting and even curative treatments.

The study of epigenetics adds another layer of complexity to our understanding of genetic factors. Epigenetics examines how gene expression is regulated by chemical modifications to DNA and histone proteins, without altering the underlying DNA sequence. These modifications can be influenced by environmental factors, such as diet, stress, and exposure to toxins, and can be passed down to subsequent generations. Epigenetic changes can activate or silence genes, affecting an individual's development and health. For example, epigenetic modifications have been implicated in cancer, where abnormal gene expression leads to uncontrolled cell growth.

The exploration of genetic factors continues to evolve, driven by advancements in technology and a deeper understanding of the human genome. The Human Genome Project, completed in 2003,

mapped the entire human genome, providing a
reference for identifying genetic variations and
understanding their functions. Ongoing research
aims to decipher the roles of non-coding regions of
the genome, which make up the majority of our
DNA and are involved in regulating gene expression
and maintaining genomic stability.

Lifestyle and Behavioral Risks

Lifestyle and behavioral risks significantly impact our
health and overall well-being. These risks are shaped
by our daily habits, choices, and environments, and
they can either promote longevity and vitality or lead
to chronic diseases and premature death.
Understanding and mitigating these risks requires a
comprehensive approach that considers various
aspects of life, from diet and physical activity to
stress management and substance use.

One of the most critical lifestyle factors influencing
health is diet. A balanced diet, rich in fruits,
vegetables, whole grains, lean proteins, and healthy
fats, provides essential nutrients that support bodily
functions and prevent diseases. Conversely, diets
high in processed foods, sugars, and unhealthy fats
contribute to obesity, heart disease, diabetes, and
other chronic conditions. The Mediterranean diet,
for instance, emphasizes plant-based foods, healthy

fats like olive oil, and lean proteins such as fish, and has been associated with reduced risks of cardiovascular diseases and improved longevity.

Physical activity is another cornerstone of a healthy lifestyle. Regular exercise strengthens the cardiovascular system, enhances muscular strength and flexibility, and supports mental health. The World Health Organization recommends at least 150 minutes of moderate-intensity aerobic activity or 75 minutes of vigorous-intensity activity per week for adults. Despite these guidelines, sedentary lifestyles have become increasingly common, exacerbated by modern conveniences and work environments that require prolonged sitting. Incorporating physical activity into daily routines, such as walking or cycling to work, taking the stairs, or engaging in recreational sports, can counteract the detrimental effects of sedentary behavior.

Stress management is crucial for maintaining mental and physical health. Chronic stress triggers a cascade of physiological responses, including the release of cortisol, which can lead to inflammation, weakened immune function, and increased risk of chronic diseases. Effective stress management techniques include mindfulness meditation, deep breathing exercises, yoga, and maintaining strong social connections. These practices help reduce stress levels, improve emotional resilience, and promote a sense of well-being.

Sleep is often an overlooked aspect of a healthy lifestyle, yet it is fundamental to overall health. Quality sleep supports cognitive function, emotional regulation, and physical health. Sleep deprivation, on the other hand, is linked to a myriad of health issues, including obesity, cardiovascular disease, diabetes, and impaired immune function. Adults typically need seven to nine hours of sleep per night, although individual needs may vary. Establishing a consistent sleep routine, creating a restful sleep environment, and avoiding stimulants like caffeine and electronic devices before bedtime can improve sleep quality.

Substance use, including tobacco, alcohol, and recreational drugs, poses significant health risks. Smoking is a leading cause of preventable death worldwide, contributing to lung cancer, heart disease, stroke, and respiratory illnesses. Quitting smoking, even later in life, can dramatically reduce these risks and improve health outcomes. Alcohol consumption, while socially accepted in many cultures, should be moderated. Excessive alcohol intake is associated with liver disease, certain cancers, and mental health disorders. The guidelines suggest that men limit alcohol to two drinks per day, and women to one drink per day. Recreational drug use, depending on the substance, can lead to addiction, mental health issues, and severe physical health consequences. Seeking support and treatment for substance abuse can significantly improve an individual's quality of life and health outcomes.

Another crucial aspect of lifestyle and behavioral risks is the role of preventive healthcare. Regular medical check-ups, vaccinations, and screenings for conditions such as hypertension, diabetes, and cancers can detect problems early, when they are most treatable. Adherence to prescribed medications and treatment plans for chronic conditions is also vital in managing health risks and preventing complications.

Social determinants of health, including socioeconomic status, education, and access to healthcare, significantly influence lifestyle and behavioral risks. Individuals in lower socioeconomic brackets often face barriers to healthy living, such as limited access to nutritious foods, safe exercise environments, and healthcare services. Addressing these disparities requires public health initiatives and policies aimed at improving education, economic opportunities, and access to healthcare for all populations.

Mental health is deeply interconnected with lifestyle and behavioral risks. Conditions such as depression, anxiety, and chronic stress can lead to unhealthy behaviors, including poor diet, physical inactivity, and substance abuse. Conversely, engaging in healthy lifestyle practices can enhance mental health. Physical activity, for instance, has been shown to reduce symptoms of depression and anxiety, while social interactions and supportive relationships can provide emotional stability and resilience.

Technology has a dual role in lifestyle and behavioral risks. On one hand, it contributes to sedentary behaviors and sleep disturbances. On the other hand, digital health tools, such as fitness trackers, mobile health apps, and telemedicine, can promote healthy behaviors and improve access to healthcare. Utilizing technology mindfully can help individuals monitor their health, set and achieve fitness goals, and access medical advice and support remotely.

Environmental factors also play a significant role in shaping lifestyle and behavioral risks. Urban design, for example, influences physical activity levels by determining the availability of parks, sidewalks, and bike lanes. Pollution and exposure to toxins can impact respiratory and cardiovascular health. Creating healthy environments through policies that promote clean air, water, and safe public spaces is essential for reducing health risks and supporting healthy lifestyles.

Behavioral change is often challenging, requiring motivation, support, and sustained effort. Understanding the psychology of behavior change can aid in developing effective strategies. The transtheoretical model, or stages of change, outlines a process through which individuals move from precontemplation to contemplation, preparation, action, and maintenance of healthy behaviors. Interventions that are tailored to an individual's stage of change, combined with support from healthcare providers, family, and community, can enhance the likelihood of successful and lasting lifestyle changes.

Education and awareness are foundational to mitigating lifestyle and behavioral risks. Public health campaigns, school programs, and community initiatives that educate individuals about healthy behaviors and the risks associated with unhealthy ones can empower people to make informed choices. Knowledge alone is not sufficient, however; creating supportive environments and policies that facilitate healthy choices is equally important.

Environmental Influences

Environmental influences play a significant role in shaping our health, behaviors, and quality of life. These influences encompass a wide range of factors, from the physical and built environments to social and economic conditions. Understanding how these elements interact with our daily lives provides valuable insights into how we can create healthier, more supportive living conditions.

The physical environment includes natural elements like air, water, and soil quality, as well as climate and weather patterns. Clean air is essential for respiratory health, yet air pollution remains a pervasive problem, particularly in urban and industrial areas. Pollutants such as particulate matter, nitrogen dioxide, and sulfur dioxide can exacerbate conditions like asthma and bronchitis and contribute to cardiovascular diseases. Efforts to reduce air pollution, such as implementing stricter emissions standards and promoting renewable energy sources, are crucial for improving public health.

Water quality is another critical aspect of the physical environment. Access to clean, safe drinking water is fundamental to human health. Contaminants like lead, arsenic, and pathogens can cause severe health issues, ranging from gastrointestinal illnesses to neurological disorders. Ensuring that water sources are protected and properly treated is vital. Additionally, maintaining infrastructure for sewage and waste management helps prevent the contamination of water supplies and reduces the spread of waterborne diseases.

Soil quality affects the food we consume, influencing nutritional content and safety. Soil contaminated with heavy metals, pesticides, or industrial waste can lead to the accumulation of harmful substances in crops, posing risks to human health. Sustainable agricultural practices, such as crop rotation, organic farming, and reduced use of chemical fertilizers and pesticides, can improve soil health and food safety. Supporting local and organic food systems also promotes environmental sustainability and reduces the carbon footprint associated with long-distance food transportation.

Climate and weather patterns have profound effects on health and well-being. Extreme weather events, such as heatwaves, floods, and hurricanes, can cause immediate physical harm and long-term health impacts. Heatwaves, for instance, increase the risk of heat-related illnesses, particularly among vulnerable populations like the elderly and those with pre-existing health conditions. Floods can lead to injuries, waterborne diseases, and mental health issues due to displacement and loss of property. Mitigating the impacts of climate change through policies that reduce greenhouse gas emissions and enhance community resilience is essential for protecting public health.

The built environment, which includes our homes, workplaces, schools, and public spaces, significantly influences our health behaviors and outcomes. Urban design and infrastructure play crucial roles in determining physical activity levels. Neighborhoods with parks, sidewalks, and bike lanes encourage walking, cycling, and outdoor activities, promoting physical fitness and reducing the risk of chronic diseases like obesity and diabetes. Conversely, areas lacking these amenities often see higher rates of sedentary behavior and related health issues.

Housing quality is another important aspect of the built environment. Poor housing conditions, such as inadequate ventilation, mold, and pest infestations, can lead to respiratory problems, allergies, and other health concerns. Overcrowding and lack of privacy can contribute to stress and mental health issues. Ensuring access to safe, affordable, and healthy housing is a key component of public health strategies. Policies that support housing improvements and provide assistance to low-income families can make a significant difference in overall health outcomes.

Workplaces also shape health through physical conditions and social dynamics. Ergonomic design, ventilation, and lighting affect physical health and productivity, while workplace culture and policies influence mental well-being. Employers can promote health by providing safe working conditions, encouraging regular breaks, and supporting mental health initiatives. Flexible work arrangements and opportunities for professional development also contribute to job satisfaction and overall well-being.

Schools are critical environments for shaping the health and behaviors of children and adolescents. Access to nutritious meals, safe recreational spaces, and health education programs can establish lifelong healthy habits. Schools that promote physical activity, provide mental health support, and create inclusive and supportive environments contribute to the overall development and well-being of students. Engaging parents and communities in school health initiatives further reinforces positive behaviors and outcomes.

The social environment encompasses relationships, community dynamics, and cultural norms. Social support networks, including family, friends, and community organizations, play a vital role in mental and emotional health. Strong social connections provide emotional support, reduce stress, and enhance resilience. Communities that foster social cohesion and provide opportunities for social interaction and engagement contribute to the well-being of their members.

Economic conditions, such as income, employment, and education, are powerful determinants of health. Socioeconomic disparities can lead to unequal access to resources, healthcare, and opportunities. Individuals in lower socioeconomic brackets often face greater health risks due to limited access to nutritious food, safe housing, and quality healthcare.

Addressing these disparities through policies that promote economic equity, access to education, and job opportunities is crucial for improving public health.

Access to healthcare services is a fundamental aspect of the social environment. Timely and affordable access to medical care, preventive services, and health education can prevent and manage diseases effectively. Health systems that prioritize equity and provide comprehensive care to all individuals, regardless of socioeconomic status, contribute to better health outcomes and reduced health disparities.

Cultural norms and practices also influence health behaviors. Cultural attitudes towards diet, physical activity, substance use, and healthcare can shape individual choices and health outcomes. Understanding and respecting cultural diversity in health promotion efforts can enhance their effectiveness. Culturally tailored interventions that consider the beliefs, practices, and preferences of different populations can improve engagement and adherence to healthy behaviors.

Environmental influences on health are complex and multifaceted, requiring a holistic and integrated approach to address them effectively. Collaboration among governments, communities, healthcare providers, and individuals is essential for creating environments that support health and well-being. Policies and initiatives that prioritize environmental sustainability, social equity, and access to resources can significantly improve public health outcomes.

Individuals can also take proactive steps to mitigate environmental influences on their health. Advocating for cleaner air and water, supporting sustainable agriculture, and participating in community planning efforts can contribute to healthier environments. Personal choices, such as reducing exposure to pollutants, engaging in physical activity, and fostering social connections, also play a role in enhancing health and well-being.

Age and Gender Considerations

Age and gender are critical factors that influence health, behavior, and social interactions. Understanding how these variables impact individuals across different stages of life and in various contexts is essential for creating effective strategies to promote well-being. This chapter delves into the unique considerations associated with age and gender, providing insights and practical advice for addressing these dimensions in a holistic manner. development is marked by distinct stages, each presenting unique physical, psychological, and social characteristics. Infants and children, for instance, require specific nutritional intake to support rapid growth and brain development. Breastfeeding is highly recommended during the first six months of life, as it provides essential nutrients and antibodies that bolster the immune system. As children grow, balanced diets rich in fruits, vegetables, whole grains, and proteins are crucial for maintaining healthy growth and development. Regular physical activity is equally important, helping to build strong bones and muscles, and fostering motor skills development.

Adolescence is a transformative period characterized by significant physical, emotional, and social changes. Puberty ushers in a cascade of hormonal changes that trigger the development of secondary sexual characteristics and reproductive capacity. Adolescents often face challenges related to body image, self-esteem, and peer pressure. Providing comprehensive sexual education, promoting healthy eating habits, and encouraging physical activity can help adolescents navigate this critical stage. Mental health support is also vital, as many mental health issues emerge during adolescence. Open communication with trusted adults and access to mental health resources can make a significant difference.

Young adulthood is typically a time of exploration, independence, and establishing lifelong habits. During this stage, individuals often make important decisions regarding education, career, relationships, and lifestyle. Encouraging healthy habits, such as regular exercise, balanced nutrition, and stress management, can lay the foundation for long-term well-being. Regular health check-ups and screenings are also important for early detection and prevention of potential health issues. Additionally, fostering supportive social networks can enhance mental health and resilience.

Middle adulthood often involves balancing multiple responsibilities, such as career, family, and personal health. This period may bring increased risk of chronic conditions like hypertension, diabetes, and cardiovascular diseases. Prioritizing preventive healthcare, maintaining a balanced diet, and staying physically active are crucial for managing these risks. Stress management techniques, such as mindfulness, yoga, and hobbies, can help mitigate the effects of stress associated with work and family life. Social connections remain important, providing emotional support and enhancing overall well-being.

Older adulthood presents its own set of challenges and opportunities. Aging is accompanied by physiological changes, such as decreased bone density, muscle mass, and cognitive function. However, many of these changes can be managed or mitigated through lifestyle choices. Engaging in regular physical activity, such as walking, swimming, or strength training, can help maintain mobility and strength. A diet rich in calcium, vitamin D, and other essential nutrients supports bone health. Mental stimulation, through activities like reading, puzzles, and social engagement, can help preserve cognitive function. Access to healthcare and social support is crucial for maintaining quality of life in older adulthood.

Gender plays a significant role in shaping health experiences and outcomes. Biological differences, such as hormonal variations, influence susceptibility to certain conditions and responses to treatments. For example, women are at higher risk of developing osteoporosis due to lower bone density and hormonal changes during menopause. Regular weight-bearing exercise, adequate calcium and vitamin D intake, and bone density screenings are essential preventive measures for women.

Men, on the other hand, are more prone to conditions like cardiovascular diseases and certain cancers. Encouraging regular physical activity, a heart-healthy diet, and routine health screenings can help mitigate these risks. Men may also benefit from education and awareness campaigns that address health issues specific to their gender, such as prostate health and mental health.

Social and cultural norms related to gender can also impact health behaviors and access to care.

Traditional gender roles and expectations may influence how individuals perceive and prioritize their health. For instance, men may be less likely to seek help for mental health issues due to societal expectations of stoicism and self-reliance. Promoting a culture that values and supports mental health for all genders can help break down these barriers and encourage individuals to seek the care they need.

Women often bear a disproportionate burden of caregiving responsibilities, which can impact their physical and mental health. Balancing caregiving with work and personal health can be challenging. Support systems, such as family leave policies, flexible work arrangements, and social support networks, can help alleviate some of these pressures. Encouraging women to prioritize self-care and seek support when needed is essential for maintaining their health and well-being.

Healthcare providers play a critical role in addressing age and gender considerations. Providing patient-centered care that takes into account the unique needs and preferences of individuals based on their age and gender can enhance health outcomes. This includes offering tailored advice, screenings, and interventions that are relevant to specific life stages and gender-related health risks.

Education and awareness campaigns can also promote understanding and action on age and gender-related health issues. Public health initiatives that target specific populations, such as adolescent health programs, women's health campaigns, and men's health awareness, can provide valuable information and resources. Community-based programs that foster social connections and support can also enhance health and well-being across different age groups and genders.

Individuals can take proactive steps to address age and gender considerations in their health journeys. Staying informed about age-appropriate health recommendations, seeking regular medical advice, and adopting healthy lifestyle habits are fundamental. Engaging in open conversations with healthcare providers about specific needs and concerns can lead to more personalized and effective care.

Preventive Measures

Preventive measures are the cornerstone of maintaining health and well-being, offering strategies to avert the onset of diseases and complications. These measures encompass a wide array of practices, from lifestyle choices and vaccinations to regular screenings and health education. Understanding and implementing these measures can significantly enhance quality of life and reduce healthcare costs.

One of the most effective preventive measures is the adoption of a healthy lifestyle. A balanced diet, rich in fruits, vegetables, whole grains, lean proteins, and healthy fats, provides the necessary nutrients to support bodily functions and prevent chronic diseases. Reducing the intake of processed foods, sugary beverages, and excessive salt is crucial for maintaining heart health, managing weight, and preventing conditions like diabetes and hypertension. Hydration is equally important, with water being the best choice to keep the body functioning optimally.

Physical activity is another vital component of a healthy lifestyle. Regular exercise helps maintain a healthy weight, strengthens muscles and bones, improves cardiovascular health, and boosts mental well-being. It is recommended to engage in at least 150 minutes of moderate-intensity aerobic activity or 75 minutes of vigorous-intensity activity each week, along with muscle-strengthening activities on two or more days a week. Finding enjoyable activities, whether it be walking, cycling, swimming, or dancing, can increase adherence to exercise routines.

Sleep is often overlooked but is essential for health. Adults generally need 7-9 hours of sleep per night to function optimally. Quality sleep supports cognitive function, mood regulation, and physical health. Establishing a regular sleep schedule, creating a restful environment, and avoiding stimulants like caffeine and electronics before bedtime can improve sleep quality. For those struggling with sleep issues, consulting a healthcare provider can help identify underlying causes and appropriate treatments.

Vaccinations are a powerful tool in preventing infectious diseases. Immunizations protect individuals and communities by reducing the spread of diseases such as measles, influenza, and HPV. Keeping up to date with recommended vaccines for different life stages, including childhood immunizations, annual flu shots, and vaccines for older adults, is crucial. Healthcare providers can offer guidance on the appropriate vaccination schedule based on individual health status and risk factors.

Regular health screenings and check-ups are essential for early detection and prevention of diseases. Routine screenings, such as blood pressure checks, cholesterol tests, and cancer screenings (e.g., mammograms, Pap smears, colonoscopies), can identify health issues before they become severe. Early detection often allows for more effective and less invasive treatments. It's important to follow the screening recommendations based on age, gender, family history, and personal health risk factors. Discussing these with a healthcare provider can help tailor a screening schedule to individual needs.

Personal hygiene practices play a significant role in preventing illness. Regular handwashing with soap and water, especially before eating and after using the restroom, can prevent the spread of infectious diseases. Oral hygiene, including brushing and flossing teeth daily and regular dental check-ups, is essential for preventing dental diseases and maintaining overall health. Proper food handling and storage practices also help prevent foodborne illnesses.

Mental health is an integral part of overall well-being, and preventive measures in this area are equally important. Stress management techniques, such as mindfulness, meditation, deep breathing exercises, and engaging in hobbies, can help reduce stress levels. Building and maintaining strong social connections provide emotional support and improve mental health. Seeking professional help when experiencing mental health issues, such as anxiety or depression, is crucial for early intervention and effective management.

Substance abuse prevention is another critical aspect of maintaining health. Avoiding tobacco use, limiting alcohol consumption, and refraining from illicit drug use can prevent numerous health issues, including respiratory diseases, liver disease, and addiction. Education and awareness programs can inform individuals about the risks associated with substance abuse and provide resources for those seeking to quit or reduce their use.

Environmental factors also play a role in preventive health measures. Reducing exposure to pollutants, such as tobacco smoke, chemicals, and heavy metals, helps prevent respiratory and other health issues. Using protective equipment, such as masks and gloves, when handling hazardous materials, and ensuring proper ventilation in living and working spaces, can mitigate health risks. Advocating for and supporting environmental policies that reduce pollution and promote clean air and water contribute to broader public health efforts.

Health education and awareness are foundational to preventive measures. Staying informed about health risks and preventive strategies empowers individuals to make informed decisions about their health. Public health campaigns, community programs, and educational resources provided by healthcare organizations can raise awareness and promote healthy behaviors. Schools and workplaces can also play a role by integrating health education into their programs.

Preventive measures are not only about individual actions but also about creating supportive environments. Policies and community initiatives that promote healthy lifestyles, such as creating safe spaces for physical activity, providing access to healthy foods, and ensuring affordable healthcare, are crucial. Employers can support preventive health by offering wellness programs, promoting work-life balance, and creating a healthy work environment.

Access to healthcare is a fundamental aspect of preventive health. Ensuring that individuals have access to primary care services, preventive screenings, vaccinations, and health education is essential for effective prevention. Health insurance coverage plays a significant role in access to these services. Advocating for policies that expand healthcare access and reduce barriers to care can improve public health outcomes.

Family and community support are vital in promoting preventive measures. Families can encourage healthy habits by cooking nutritious meals together, engaging in physical activities, and supporting each other's health goals. Community groups and organizations can provide resources, support networks, and programs that promote health and well-being. Volunteering and participating in community health initiatives can also foster a sense of purpose and connection.

Technology can be a valuable tool in preventive health. Wearable devices and mobile apps that track physical activity, diet, sleep, and other health metrics can help individuals monitor their health and make informed decisions. Telehealth services provide convenient access to healthcare providers for consultations, follow-ups, and health advice. Online resources and health information platforms can offer educational materials and support for preventive health practices.

Chapter 4

Diagnostic Tools in Cardiology

Physical Examination and History Taking

A thorough physical examination and comprehensive history taking are fundamental components of medical practice, providing invaluable insights into a patient's health status. These processes are not merely routine procedures but critical steps that build the foundation for accurate diagnosis and effective treatment plans. By meticulously gathering a patient's medical history and conducting a detailed physical examination, healthcare providers can identify potential health issues early, understand the context of presenting symptoms, and establish a rapport essential for ongoing care.

The process begins with history taking, which involves collecting detailed information about the patient's past and present health. This conversation is more than a series of questions; it is an opportunity to understand the patient's story, concerns, and health goals. Effective history taking requires excellent communication skills, empathy, and the ability to listen actively.

First, the patient's chief complaint, or the primary reason for the visit, is identified. This typically involves asking open-ended questions like, "What brings you in today?" to encourage the patient to describe their symptoms in their own words. This initial information sets the stage for a more detailed exploration of the issue at hand.

Following the chief complaint, a detailed history of the present illness is obtained. This includes the onset, duration, and progression of symptoms, along with any factors that exacerbate or alleviate the condition. Questions about associated symptoms, previous episodes, and any treatments already tried provide a comprehensive picture of the current health issue.

The patient's past medical history is also crucial. This encompasses previous illnesses, surgeries, hospitalizations, and any ongoing medical conditions. Information about allergies and current medications, including over-the-counter drugs and supplements, is essential to avoid potential drug interactions and allergic reactions. Immunization status should also be reviewed to ensure the patient is up to date with recommended vaccines.

A family history offers insights into genetic predispositions to certain conditions. By asking about the health of immediate family members, including parents, siblings, and children, healthcare providers can identify patterns that may suggest a hereditary risk for diseases such as diabetes, heart disease, or certain cancers.

Social history provides context about the patient's lifestyle and environment, which can significantly impact health. This includes information about occupation, living conditions, dietary habits, physical activity, substance use (such as tobacco, alcohol, and recreational drugs), and social support systems. Understanding these factors can help tailor recommendations and interventions to the patient's specific circumstances.

A review of systems involves a systematic inquiry about symptoms related to different body systems, from head to toe. This comprehensive approach ensures that no potential issues are overlooked and helps to corroborate findings from the physical examination.

With a detailed history in hand, the physical examination begins. This process is both an art and a science, requiring keen observation, palpation, percussion, and auscultation skills. Each step of the examination provides vital information about the patient's physical condition.

The general survey offers an initial impression of the patient's overall health. Observations about the patient's appearance, including level of consciousness, distress, mobility, posture, and hygiene, can provide important clues. Vital signs—temperature, pulse, respiration, blood pressure, and sometimes oxygen saturation—are measured to assess basic physiological functions.

The examination proceeds systematically, typically starting from the head and moving down to the feet. The head and neck examination includes inspecting the scalp, face, eyes, ears, nose, mouth, and throat. Palpating lymph nodes, thyroid gland, and examining the range of motion in the neck can identify abnormalities.

The chest examination focuses on the heart and lungs. Auscultation with a stethoscope allows for the assessment of heart sounds, murmurs, and breath sounds. Percussion and palpation help evaluate the size, consistency, and presence of any abnormalities. Observing respiratory effort and symmetry of chest movements is also crucial.

The abdominal examination involves inspection, auscultation, percussion, and palpation to assess the organs within the abdominal cavity. This can reveal issues such as organ enlargement, masses, or fluid accumulation. Listening to bowel sounds can provide information about gastrointestinal function.

Examination of the musculoskeletal system includes evaluating the joints, muscles, and bones. This involves assessing the range of motion, strength, and any signs of inflammation or deformity. Observing gait and posture can also provide insights into musculoskeletal health.

The neurological examination assesses the central and peripheral nervous systems. This includes evaluating mental status, cranial nerves, motor and sensory function, reflexes, coordination, and balance. Detailed neurological testing can help localize lesions and determine the extent of neurological impairment.

Throughout the examination, it is essential to maintain a respectful and sensitive approach, ensuring the patient's comfort and dignity. Explaining each step of the process and seeking consent before performing more intimate or potentially uncomfortable procedures is crucial for building trust.

Once the history and physical examination are complete, the findings are synthesized to develop a differential diagnosis. This list of potential conditions considers the most likely causes based on the patient's symptoms, history, and physical examination findings. Additional diagnostic tests, such as laboratory tests or imaging studies, may be ordered to narrow down the diagnosis and confirm the suspected condition.

Effective documentation of the history and physical examination is essential. Clear, concise, and accurate records ensure continuity of care and provide a reference for future visits. These records also facilitate communication with other healthcare providers involved in the patient's care.

The information gathered during history taking and physical examination is integral to developing a personalized care plan. This plan addresses the patient's immediate health concerns and includes preventive measures, lifestyle modifications, and follow-up care. Educating the patient about their condition and involving them in decision-making fosters a collaborative approach to health management.

Blood Tests and Biomarkers

Blood tests and biomarkers are essential tools in modern medicine, offering critical insights into a patient's health status, diagnosing diseases, monitoring treatment efficacy, and predicting medical outcomes. The ability to measure various substances in the blood allows healthcare providers to detect abnormalities and make informed decisions about patient care. Understanding the types, purposes, and interpretations of these tests can empower patients and enhance the effectiveness of medical interventions.

The complete blood count (CBC) is one of the most commonly ordered blood tests. It provides a broad overview of a patient's general health and can help detect a range of disorders, including infections, anemia, and leukemia. The CBC measures several components of blood, including red blood cells (RBCs), white blood cells (WBCs), hemoglobin, hematocrit, and platelets. Each component gives specific information: RBCs indicate oxygen-carrying capacity, WBCs point to immune function, hemoglobin and hematocrit offer insights into blood's oxygen-carrying capacity, and platelets are crucial for blood clotting.

A comprehensive metabolic panel (CMP) is another standard test that evaluates overall health and screens for diseases. The CMP includes tests for blood glucose, calcium, electrolytes (such as sodium and potassium), and kidney and liver function. Abnormal levels can indicate issues like diabetes, kidney disease, or liver dysfunction. For instance, elevated blood glucose levels may suggest diabetes or prediabetes, while abnormal calcium levels can indicate problems with the parathyroid glands or bone diseases.

Lipid panels are crucial for assessing cardiovascular health. They measure levels of cholesterol and triglycerides in the blood. The panel typically includes total cholesterol, low-density lipoprotein (LDL) cholesterol, high-density lipoprotein (HDL) cholesterol, and triglycerides. LDL cholesterol, often referred to as "bad" cholesterol, can lead to plaque buildup in arteries, increasing the risk of heart disease and stroke. Conversely, HDL cholesterol, or "good" cholesterol, helps remove LDL cholesterol from the bloodstream. Balancing these lipid levels through diet, exercise, and medication can significantly reduce cardiovascular risk.

Liver function tests (LFTs) assess the health of the liver by measuring levels of proteins, liver enzymes, and bilirubin in the blood. Elevated levels of enzymes such as alanine transaminase (ALT) and aspartate transaminase (AST) can indicate liver damage or inflammation, potentially caused by conditions like hepatitis, fatty liver disease, or alcohol abuse. Bilirubin levels can provide insights into liver function and bile duct health, with high levels potentially indicating jaundice or bile duct obstruction.

Kidney function tests measure levels of waste products in the blood, including blood urea nitrogen (BUN) and creatinine, to assess how well the kidneys are filtering blood. Elevated levels of these substances can indicate kidney dysfunction or disease. The glomerular filtration rate (GFR) is another critical measure of kidney function, estimating how much blood passes through the glomeruli (tiny filters in the kidneys) each minute. A low GFR can signify chronic kidney disease.

Endocrine function tests evaluate hormone levels to diagnose and manage disorders related to the endocrine glands. For example, thyroid function tests measure levels of thyroid hormones (such as thyroxine, or T4, and triiodothyronine, or T3) and thyroid-stimulating hormone (TSH) to assess thyroid health. Abnormal levels can indicate conditions like hypothyroidism or hyperthyroidism. Similarly, hormone tests for the adrenal glands, pituitary gland, and reproductive organs can diagnose disorders such as Addison's disease, Cushing's syndrome, and polycystic ovary syndrome (PCOS).

Inflammatory markers, such as C-reactive protein (CRP) and erythrocyte sedimentation rate (ESR), help detect inflammation in the body. Elevated levels of these markers can indicate acute or chronic inflammatory conditions, such as infections, autoimmune diseases, or cancers. While these markers are nonspecific, meaning they do not pinpoint the exact cause of inflammation, they are valuable for monitoring disease activity and response to treatment.

Blood tests for infectious diseases detect the presence of pathogens like bacteria, viruses, fungi, or parasites. These tests can identify infections such as HIV, hepatitis, and tuberculosis. Polymerase chain reaction (PCR) tests detect the genetic material of pathogens, providing accurate and rapid diagnosis. Serology tests measure antibodies or antigens in the blood, indicating current or past infections. These tests are crucial for disease surveillance, outbreak control, and guiding appropriate treatment.

Tumor markers are substances produced by cancer cells or by the body in response to cancer. Measuring these markers in the blood can help diagnose and monitor certain types of cancer. For instance, prostate-specific antigen (PSA) is a marker for prostate cancer, while cancer antigen 125 (CA-125) is used in ovarian cancer diagnosis and monitoring. Although tumor markers are not definitive for cancer diagnosis, they provide valuable information for assessing disease progression and treatment response.

Genetic testing analyzes DNA to identify genetic mutations or variations associated with inherited disorders. Blood samples can be used to detect conditions such as cystic fibrosis, sickle cell anemia, and BRCA gene mutations linked to increased breast and ovarian cancer risk. Genetic testing can also guide personalized treatment plans, predict disease risk, and inform family planning decisions.

Interpreting blood test results requires understanding reference ranges, which indicate the normal levels of each measured substance. Results outside these ranges may suggest an underlying health issue. However, it is essential to consider factors such as age, sex, medical history, and medications when interpreting results, as these can influence normal ranges and test outcomes.

Regular blood testing is a proactive approach to health management. Routine screenings can detect potential health issues before they become symptomatic, allowing for early intervention and better outcomes. For individuals with chronic conditions, regular monitoring helps manage the disease and adjust treatment plans as needed. Communicating openly with healthcare providers about test results and their implications ensures that patients are informed and engaged in their health care.

While blood tests are powerful diagnostic tools, they are not without limitations. False positives and false negatives can occur, and abnormal results may require additional testing for confirmation. It is also crucial to consider the whole clinical picture, as test results should be interpreted in the context of the patient's symptoms, history, and other diagnostic findings.

Electrocardiogram (ECG)

The room was filled with the steady hum of the ECG machine, a background symphony that many patients found oddly comforting. An electrocardiogram (ECG) is a pivotal diagnostic tool in the realm of cardiovascular medicine. It provides a window into the heart's electrical activity, helping to diagnose a myriad of cardiac conditions, from arrhythmias to myocardial infarctions. Understanding the function, procedure, and interpretation of an ECG is crucial for both healthcare providers and patients.

An ECG measures the electrical impulses that prompt the heart to beat. These impulses are generated in the sinoatrial (SA) node, often referred to as the heart's natural pacemaker. The SA node sends out an electrical signal that travels through the atria, causing them to contract and push blood into the ventricles. The signal then passes through the atrioventricular (AV) node, which acts as a gatekeeper, slowing the signal before it moves to the ventricles. This delay allows the ventricles to fill with blood before they contract and send blood to the lungs and the rest of the body.

The ECG machine records this electrical activity through electrodes placed on the skin. Typically, ten electrodes are used: one on each limb and six across the chest. These electrodes detect the tiny electrical changes on the skin that arise from the heart muscle's electrophysiologic pattern of depolarizing and repolarizing during each heartbeat. The recorded data is presented as a graph, with the horizontal axis representing time and the vertical axis representing voltage. The resulting waveform, known as an electrocardiogram, consists of several distinct parts: the P wave, QRS complex, T wave, and sometimes a U wave.

Reading an ECG might seem daunting at first, but breaking it down into its component parts makes it more manageable. The P wave represents atrial depolarization, the process that triggers the atria to contract. It is usually a small, rounded wave that precedes the larger QRS complex. The QRS complex, a rapid sequence of three deflections, represents ventricular depolarization and is much larger than the P wave due to the greater muscle mass of the ventricles. Following the QRS complex, the T wave represents ventricular repolarization, the recovery phase when the ventricles prepare for the next beat. Occasionally, a U wave may follow the T wave, though its exact significance remains a topic of debate among cardiologists.

Interpreting an ECG requires a systematic approach. First, healthcare providers assess the heart rate by counting the number of QRS complexes in a given time frame, typically 6 seconds, and multiplying by 10 to get the beats per minute. A normal resting heart rate for adults ranges from 60 to 100 beats per minute. Next, the rhythm is examined to determine if it is regular or irregular. The regularity of the rhythm is assessed by measuring the intervals between consecutive R waves.

The ECG is also scrutinized for the presence of any abnormal waves or complexes that could indicate underlying cardiac issues. For instance, a prolonged PR interval (the time between the start of the P wave and the start of the QRS complex) might suggest a first-degree atrioventricular block, a condition where the electrical conduction between the atria and ventricles is delayed. An elevated ST segment (the flat section of the ECG between the end of the S wave and the start of the T wave) can be a sign of myocardial infarction, commonly known as a heart attack, whereas a depressed ST segment might indicate myocardial ischemia, a condition where blood flow to the heart muscle is reduced.

The interpretation of an ECG is not limited to identifying heart rate and rhythm abnormalities. It also plays a crucial role in diagnosing and managing various cardiac conditions. For example, atrial fibrillation, a common arrhythmia characterized by disorganized electrical activity in the atria, is diagnosed by the absence of distinct P waves and the presence of an irregularly irregular rhythm. Ventricular tachycardia, a potentially life-threatening condition where the ventricles beat very quickly, can be identified by a series of wide QRS complexes.

In addition to arrhythmias, an ECG can help diagnose structural heart diseases and electrolyte imbalances. Left ventricular hypertrophy, a condition where the muscle wall of the heart's left ventricle thickens, often due to high blood pressure, can be suggested by specific changes in the QRS complex. Hyperkalemia, an elevated level of potassium in the blood, can cause characteristic ECG changes, such as peaked T waves and widening of the QRS complex.

While an ECG is a powerful diagnostic tool, it is important to recognize its limitations. It provides a snapshot of the heart's electrical activity at a single point in time and may not capture intermittent abnormalities. Therefore, if a patient experiences symptoms such as palpitations or chest pain that are not present during the ECG recording, additional tests like Holter monitoring or an event recorder might be necessary. These devices record the heart's activity over an extended period, increasing the likelihood of detecting transient abnormalities.

The utility of an ECG extends beyond diagnosis. It is also instrumental in guiding treatment decisions and monitoring the effectiveness of interventions. For instance, in patients with pacemakers, ECGs can verify proper functioning of the device. In those receiving antiarrhythmic medications, ECGs can help assess the drug's efficacy and detect any adverse effects, such as QT interval prolongation, which can predispose to dangerous arrhythmias.

Moreover, an ECG is a valuable tool in preventive cardiology. Routine ECGs can identify individuals at risk of developing cardiovascular diseases, enabling early interventions that can mitigate risk factors. For example, an ECG might reveal signs of left ventricular hypertrophy in a patient with hypertension, prompting more aggressive blood pressure management to prevent complications like heart failure.

Understanding the emotional and psychological impact of an ECG on patients is also essential. The experience of undergoing an ECG can evoke anxiety, particularly if the patient is already concerned about their heart health. Clear communication and education about the procedure and its purpose can alleviate fears and foster a sense of collaboration between the patient and healthcare provider. Ensuring that patients understand their ECG results and the subsequent steps in their care plan enhances their engagement and adherence to treatment.

In the broader context of healthcare, the accessibility and non-invasiveness of ECGs make them an invaluable resource in diverse settings, from primary care clinics to emergency departments. Portable ECG machines and advancements in telemedicine have further expanded the reach of this diagnostic tool, allowing for remote monitoring and consultations. This is particularly beneficial in underserved areas, where access to specialized cardiac care might be limited.

Echocardiography

The gentle whir of the echocardiography machine filled the examination room, blending with the rhythmic beeping of the heart rate monitor. For many patients, the experience of undergoing an echocardiogram is both reassuring and enlightening. Echocardiography, often referred to as an "echo," is a vital imaging technique in cardiology that uses ultrasound waves to create detailed images of the heart. This non-invasive procedure provides invaluable insights into the heart's structure and function, aiding in the diagnosis and management of various cardiovascular conditions.

The journey of echocardiography begins with the transducer, a small handheld device that emits high-frequency sound waves. When placed on the chest, the transducer sends these sound waves through the body. As the waves encounter different tissues, they bounce back to the transducer, which then translates them into images displayed on a monitor. This real-time visualization allows healthcare providers to observe the heart's chambers, valves, walls, and blood flow, providing a comprehensive assessment of cardiac health.

One of the primary advantages of echocardiography is its ability to produce dynamic images of the heart. Unlike static imaging techniques, such as X-rays, an echo captures the heart in motion, offering a live view of its beating. This capability is crucial for evaluating heart function and detecting abnormalities that might not be apparent in still images. For instance, echocardiography can reveal the motion of the heart walls, the opening and closing of valves, and the flow of blood through the heart and major vessels.

Echocardiography comes in several forms, each tailored to specific diagnostic needs. Transthoracic echocardiography (TTE) is the most common type, involving the placement of the transducer on the outside of the chest. This method is quick, painless, and highly effective for most patients. In cases where more detailed images are needed, transesophageal echocardiography (TEE) may be used. TEE involves passing a specialized transducer down the esophagus, providing closer proximity to the heart and clearer images, especially of the posterior structures. Stress echocardiography, another variant, combines ultrasound imaging with physical exercise or pharmacological agents to assess how the heart performs under stress, revealing issues that might not be evident at rest.

The application of echocardiography spans a wide range of cardiac conditions. One of its most common uses is in the evaluation of heart valve diseases. By visualizing the heart valves in action, echocardiography can identify abnormalities such as stenosis (narrowing of the valve) or regurgitation (leakage of the valve). These conditions can significantly impact heart function, leading to symptoms like shortness of breath, fatigue, and chest pain. Echocardiography not only helps in diagnosing these valve disorders but also in determining their severity and guiding treatment decisions.

Heart failure is another area where echocardiography plays a pivotal role. Heart failure, a condition where the heart cannot pump blood effectively, can arise from various underlying causes, including coronary artery disease, high blood pressure, and cardiomyopathy. Echocardiography assesses the heart's pumping ability by measuring the ejection fraction, which represents the percentage of blood pumped out of the ventricles with each heartbeat. A reduced ejection fraction indicates systolic dysfunction, a common feature of heart failure. Additionally, echocardiography can evaluate diastolic function, which refers to the heart's ability to relax and fill with blood between beats. Diastolic dysfunction, another form of heart failure, can be diagnosed through specific echo findings.

Congenital heart diseases, which are structural abnormalities present from birth, are also effectively diagnosed and monitored using echocardiography. These conditions can range from simple issues like a small hole in the heart (septal defect) to complex malformations involving multiple structures. Echocardiography provides detailed images that help delineate the anatomy and guide surgical or interventional planning. For pediatric patients, this non-invasive technique is particularly valuable as it avoids the need for more invasive procedures.

The utility of echocardiography extends to the evaluation of pericardial diseases as well. The pericardium, a thin sac surrounding the heart, can become inflamed (pericarditis) or fill with fluid (pericardial effusion), both of which can affect heart function. Echocardiography can detect pericardial effusion and assess its impact on the heart's ability to fill and pump blood. In cases of cardiac tamponade, a life-threatening condition where fluid accumulation exerts pressure on the heart, echocardiography provides critical information for timely intervention.

Echocardiography is also instrumental in the diagnosis and management of cardiomyopathies, a group of diseases that affect the heart muscle. These conditions can lead to abnormal heart structure and function, often progressing to heart failure. By visualizing the size, shape, and motion of the heart, echocardiography helps identify different types of cardiomyopathies, such as dilated cardiomyopathy, hypertrophic cardiomyopathy, and restrictive cardiomyopathy. It also aids in monitoring disease progression and the effectiveness of treatments.

In the realm of acute cardiac care, echocardiography is indispensable. In the emergency setting, it can rapidly assess patients presenting with chest pain, shortness of breath, or other symptoms suggestive of acute coronary syndrome or pulmonary embolism. Point-of-care echocardiography, performed at the bedside, provides immediate information that can guide critical decisions. For instance, in patients with suspected myocardial infarction, echocardiography can detect regional wall motion abnormalities indicative of ischemia. In cases of suspected pulmonary embolism, it can reveal right ventricular strain, a sign of increased pressure in the pulmonary arteries.

The versatility of echocardiography is further highlighted by its role in guiding interventional procedures. During catheter-based interventions, such as transcatheter aortic valve replacement (TAVR) or mitral valve repair, real-time echocardiographic imaging ensures precise placement and deployment of devices. Intracardiac echocardiography (ICE), a specialized form of echo performed from within the heart using a catheter-based transducer, provides detailed images that enhance the safety and efficacy of these procedures.

Moreover, echocardiography is a cornerstone in preventive cardiology. Routine echocardiograms can identify early signs of heart disease, even before symptoms develop. For individuals with risk factors such as hypertension, diabetes, or a family history of cardiac conditions, regular echo assessments can detect subclinical changes and prompt early intervention. This proactive approach contributes to better long-term cardiovascular outcomes.

Understanding the patient experience is crucial in echocardiography. While the procedure is generally well-tolerated, it can evoke anxiety, particularly in those undergoing it for the first time. Clear communication about what to expect and the purpose of the echo can alleviate concerns.

Explaining the process step-by-step, from the application of gel to the movement of the transducer, helps demystify the procedure. Additionally, discussing how the results will inform their care plan fosters a collaborative relationship between patients and healthcare providers.

Technological advancements continue to enhance the capabilities of echocardiography. Three-dimensional echocardiography (3D echo) provides more detailed and accurate representations of cardiac structures, improving diagnostic precision. Strain imaging, a technique that measures myocardial deformation, offers insights into subtle changes in heart function that are not apparent on conventional echocardiography. These innovations, coupled with artificial intelligence and machine learning algorithms, are poised to further revolutionize the field, enabling more sophisticated analysis and personalized care.

Advanced Imaging Techniques (CT, MRI)

Emerging from the corridors of modern medical technology, advanced imaging techniques like Computed Tomography (CT) and Magnetic Resonance Imaging (MRI) have revolutionized the landscape of diagnostic medicine. These sophisticated tools provide unparalleled insights into the human body, enabling physicians to diagnose and treat a myriad of conditions with precision and confidence.

CT and MRI, while both invaluable, differ significantly in their mechanisms and applications. CT, or Computed Tomography, harnesses the power of X-rays to produce detailed cross-sectional images of the body. By rotating around the patient, the CT scanner captures multiple X-ray images from different angles. These images are then processed by a computer to create a comprehensive, three-dimensional view of the internal structures. This ability to visualize the body in slices, much like a loaf of bread, allows for meticulous examination of bones, blood vessels, and soft tissues.

MRI, or Magnetic Resonance Imaging, operates on a different principle. Instead of X-rays, it uses powerful magnets and radio waves to generate images. The patient is placed inside a large magnet, and the magnetic field temporarily realigns hydrogen atoms in the body. Radio waves are then emitted, causing these atoms to produce signals that are detected by the MRI machine and converted into detailed images. MRI excels at visualizing soft tissues, making it particularly useful for brain, spinal cord, and joint imaging.

One of the most significant advantages of CT is its speed. A full-body CT scan can be completed in a matter of minutes, making it an excellent choice for emergency situations where time is of the essence. For instance, in cases of trauma, stroke, or suspected internal bleeding, a CT scan can quickly provide critical information that guides immediate intervention. Its ability to detect subtle differences in tissue density also makes it a powerful tool for identifying tumors, infections, and other abnormalities.

Moreover, CT angiography has become a cornerstone in vascular imaging. By injecting a contrast dye into the bloodstream, CT scans can produce detailed images of blood vessels, revealing blockages, aneurysms, and other vascular issues. This non-invasive technique has largely replaced conventional angiography, reducing the risk and discomfort for patients. Additionally, advanced CT technologies, such as dual-energy CT, offer enhanced tissue characterization and better detection of conditions like gout, renal stones, and pulmonary embolisms.

In contrast, MRI's strength lies in its exceptional contrast resolution. It provides a more detailed and nuanced view of soft tissues compared to CT. This makes MRI the modality of choice for imaging the brain and spinal cord. Neurologists rely on MRI to diagnose conditions such as multiple sclerosis, brain tumors, and neurodegenerative diseases. The ability to visualize the brain in exquisite detail helps in identifying subtle lesions, guiding treatment plans, and monitoring disease progression.

Orthopedic imaging is another area where MRI shines. It provides clear images of joints, cartilage, ligaments, and tendons, which are crucial for diagnosing sports injuries and degenerative conditions like arthritis. MRI's capability to capture multiple planes of the body without repositioning the patient adds to its versatility. For example, in cases of knee injuries, MRI can reveal tears in the meniscus or ligaments that might not be visible on other imaging modalities.

Cardiac MRI, a specialized form of MRI, offers detailed images of the heart and its structures. It is invaluable for assessing cardiac function, detecting myocardial infarction, and evaluating conditions like cardiomyopathy and congenital heart disease. Unlike CT, MRI does not expose patients to ionizing radiation, making it a safer option for repeated imaging, particularly in young patients and those requiring long-term follow-up.

The use of contrast agents enhances the diagnostic capabilities of both CT and MRI. In CT, iodine-based contrast agents are commonly used to highlight blood vessels, organs, and other structures.

In MRI, gadolinium-based contrast agents improve the visibility of abnormalities by altering the magnetic properties of nearby water molecules. However, the use of contrast agents requires careful consideration, particularly in patients with kidney dysfunction, as they can pose risks of adverse reactions.

Despite their strengths, both CT and MRI have limitations and are not without risks. CT scans expose patients to ionizing radiation, which can increase the lifetime risk of cancer, especially with repeated exposures. Therefore, the use of CT should be judicious, especially in younger patients. MRI, on the other hand, is contraindicated in patients with certain metallic implants or devices, as the strong magnetic fields can interfere with their function or cause injury. Additionally, MRI can be challenging for claustrophobic patients, although open MRI machines and sedatives can mitigate this issue.

Advancements in CT and MRI technology continue to push the boundaries of what these imaging modalities can achieve. For instance, the development of functional MRI (fMRI) has opened new frontiers in neuroscience. fMRI measures brain activity by detecting changes in blood flow, providing insights into brain function and connectivity. This has profound implications for understanding and treating neurological and psychiatric disorders.

Similarly, the advent of CT perfusion imaging has improved the assessment of blood flow in various organs, particularly the brain. In the context of acute stroke, CT perfusion imaging can identify areas of the brain that are at risk but still salvageable, guiding timely and targeted interventions. These innovations underscore the dynamic nature of imaging technology and its ongoing evolution.

In clinical practice, the choice between CT and MRI depends on multiple factors, including the clinical question, patient condition, and specific anatomical area of interest. Often, these modalities are complementary rather than competitive. For example, a patient with suspected stroke might undergo a CT scan initially to rule out hemorrhage, followed by an MRI to assess for ischemic changes. Similarly, in cancer staging, CT might be used for a quick overview of disease spread, while MRI provides detailed characterization of specific lesions.

Understanding the patient's experience during CT and MRI scans is crucial for healthcare providers. Clear communication about what to expect can alleviate anxiety and improve cooperation. For CT scans, patients should be informed about the need to remain still and the possibility of receiving a contrast injection. For MRI, explaining the nature of the loud noises and the importance of staying still can help patients feel more at ease. Providing earplugs or headphones with music can also enhance comfort during MRI exams.

The integration of advanced imaging techniques into routine practice has undoubtedly transformed patient care. By providing detailed and accurate anatomical and functional information, CT and MRI contribute to early diagnosis, precise treatment planning, and improved outcomes. As technology continues to advance, these imaging modalities will likely become even more integral to the practice of medicine, offering new possibilities for understanding and treating disease.

The evolution of CT and MRI has also highlighted the importance of interdisciplinary collaboration. Radiologists, technologists, and referring physicians must work together to ensure that the right imaging modality is chosen for each patient, that the scans are performed correctly, and that the results are interpreted accurately. This collaborative approach enhances the quality of care and maximizes the benefits of advanced imaging technologies.

Stress Testing

Stress testing is a crucial tool in evaluating the cardiovascular health of patients, particularly those with suspected or known coronary artery disease. It provides valuable information about how the heart functions under physical stress, which can reveal issues not apparent when the body is at rest. By simulating the conditions under which the heart works harder, healthcare professionals can identify problems with blood flow, heart rhythms, and overall cardiac performance.

The process typically involves monitoring the heart while the patient exercises on a treadmill or stationary bike. In some cases, when physical exercise isn't feasible, pharmacological agents are used to mimic the effects of exercise on the heart. Regardless of the method, the goal remains the same: to increase the heart's workload and observe how it responds.

One of the primary indications for stress testing is the evaluation of chest pain. When a patient presents with chest discomfort, determining whether it's related to coronary artery disease is critical. Stress testing can help differentiate between cardiac and non-cardiac causes of pain. By comparing the heart's performance during exercise to its baseline function, doctors can identify areas where blood flow might be restricted due to narrowed or blocked arteries.

Additionally, stress testing is instrumental in assessing the effectiveness of treatments in patients with known heart conditions. For those who have undergone procedures like angioplasty or coronary artery bypass grafting, stress testing can evaluate the success of these interventions. It provides a dynamic picture of heart function, helping to guide further treatment decisions and adjust medications as needed.

The procedure begins with a baseline assessment. Patients are connected to an electrocardiogram (ECG) to monitor the heart's electrical activity, and their blood pressure is taken. This establishes a benchmark of the heart's function at rest. The patient then begins exercising, with the intensity gradually increasing. Throughout the test, the ECG and blood pressure readings are continuously monitored.

One of the key measurements during stress testing is the MET, or metabolic equivalent. This quantifies the amount of energy expended during physical activity. Achieving a certain MET level is essential for diagnosing various cardiac conditions. For instance, failing to reach 5 METs might indicate a significant impairment in cardiac function, prompting further investigation.

Healthcare providers closely watch for signs of ischemia, which occurs when the heart muscle doesn't get enough oxygen-rich blood. This can manifest as changes in the ECG, such as ST-segment depression, or as symptoms like chest pain, shortness of breath, or fatigue. These signs indicate that parts of the heart may not be receiving adequate blood flow, suggesting the presence of coronary artery disease.

Stress testing isn't confined to diagnosing coronary artery disease alone. It can also detect arrhythmias that may only occur during physical exertion. Some patients might have normal heart rhythms at rest but develop irregularities like atrial fibrillation or ventricular tachycardia when their heart rate increases. Identifying these arrhythmias during stress testing allows for timely intervention and management.

Another valuable aspect of stress testing is its role in risk stratification. For patients with known heart disease, the results can help predict the likelihood of future cardiac events such as heart attacks. Those who perform poorly on stress tests or exhibit significant ischemia are at higher risk and may require more aggressive treatment and closer monitoring.

Modern advancements have enhanced the capabilities of stress testing. Stress echocardiography, for example, combines traditional stress testing with ultrasound imaging. This technique provides real-time images of the heart's structure and function during exercise, offering additional insights into how the heart copes with increased workload. It can reveal issues like wall motion abnormalities, which indicate regions of the heart that are not contracting properly due to insufficient blood flow.

Nuclear stress testing is another advanced method that involves injecting a small amount of radioactive tracer into the bloodstream. This tracer highlights areas of the heart with good blood flow versus those with reduced perfusion. Images taken before and after exercise allow doctors to compare the distribution of blood flow, pinpointing areas of concern.

While stress testing is a powerful diagnostic tool, it does have limitations. False positives and false negatives can occur, meaning the test might indicate a problem when there isn't one or miss an existing issue. Therefore, stress testing is often used in conjunction with other diagnostic methods, such as coronary angiography, to confirm findings and make definitive diagnoses.

Safety is a paramount concern during stress testing. While the procedure is generally safe, it does carry some risks, particularly for patients with severe heart conditions. Healthcare providers are trained to manage any complications that arise, such as abnormal heart rhythms or excessive blood pressure changes. Emergency equipment and medications are readily available to address these situations promptly.

Patients preparing for a stress test should follow specific guidelines to ensure accurate results. They are usually advised to avoid eating, smoking, or consuming caffeine for several hours before the test. Wearing comfortable clothing and supportive shoes is also important, as they will be exercising. It's crucial to inform the healthcare team of any medications being taken, as some drugs can affect heart rate and blood pressure, potentially altering the test results.

Understanding the patient's experience during stress testing is essential for healthcare providers. Clear communication about what to expect can alleviate anxiety and improve cooperation. Patients should know that they will be monitored continuously and that the exercise will be stopped if they experience significant discomfort or any concerning symptoms.

The information gleaned from stress testing extends beyond diagnosis. It plays a vital role in guiding treatment strategies. For instance, patients with significant ischemia identified during stress testing may benefit from revascularization procedures like angioplasty or bypass surgery. Those with less severe findings might be managed with lifestyle modifications and medications aimed at reducing cardiac risk factors.

Stress testing also has implications for lifestyle and rehabilitation. Patients who have undergone successful treatment for heart conditions can use the results from stress testing to guide their physical activity levels. Cardiac rehabilitation programs often incorporate stress testing to tailor exercise regimens that are safe and effective, promoting recovery and long-term heart health.

www.ingramcontent.com/pod-product-compliance
Lightning Source LLC
Chambersburg PA
CBHW072012150726
47999CB00002B/615